Management of Operating Room Critical Events

Editor

ALEXANDER A. HANNENBERG

ANESTHESIOLOGY CLINICS

www.anesthesiology.theclinics.com

Consulting Editor
LEE A. FLEISHER

December 2020 • Volume 38 • Number 4

ELSEVIER

1600 John F. Kennedy Boulevard • Suite 1800 • Philadelphia, Pennsylvania, 19103-2899

http://www.theclinics.com

ANESTHESIOLOGY CLINICS Volume 38, Number 4
December 2020 ISSN 1932-2275, ISBN-13: 978-0-323-76128-4

Editor: Joanna Collett
Developmental Editor: Nicholas Henderson

Anesthesiology Clinics (ISSN 1932-2275) is published quarterly by Elsevier Inc., 360 Park Avenue South, New York, NY 10010-1710. Months of issue are March, June, September, and December. Periodicals postage paid at New York, NY and at additional mailing offices. Subscription prices are $100.00 per year (US student/resident), $364.00 per year (US individuals), $446.00 per year (Canadian individuals), $728.00 per year (US institutions), $920.00 per year (Canadian institutions), $100.00 per year (Canadian student/resident), $225.00 per year (foreign student/resident), $474.00 per year (foreign individuals), and $920.00 per year (foreign institutions). To receive student and resident rate, orders must be accompanied by name of affiliated institution, date of term, and the *signature* of program/residency coordinator on institutions letterhead. Orders will be billed at individual rate until proof of status is received. Foreign air speed delivery is included in all *Clinics'* subscription prices. All prices are subject to change without notice. POSTMASTER: Send address changes to *Anesthesiology Clinics,* Elsevier Health Sciences Division, Subscription Customer Service, 3251 Riverport Lane, Maryland Heights, MO 63043. Customer Service (orders, claims, online, change of address): Elsevier Health Sciences Division, Subscription Customer Service, 3251 Riverport Lane, Maryland Heights, MO 63043. **Tel:1-800-654-2452 (U.S. and Canada); 314-447-8871 (outside U.S. and Canada). Fax: 314-447-8029. E-mail: journalscustomerservice-usa@elsevier.com (for print support); journalsonlinesupport-usa@elsevier.com (for online support).**

Reprints. For copies of 100 or more of articles in this publication, please contact the Commercial Reprints Department, Elsevier Inc., 360 Park Avenue South, New York, NY 10010-1710. Tel.: 212-633-3874; Fax: 212-633-3820; E-mail: reprints@elsevier.com.

Anesthesiology Clinics, is also published in Spanish by McGraw-Hill Inter-americana Editores S. A., P.O. Box 5-237, 06500 Mexico D. F., Mexico.

Anesthesiology Clinics, is covered in *MEDLINE/PubMed (Index Medicus), Current Contents/Clinical Medicine, Excerpta Medica, ISI/BIOMED*, and *Chemical Abstracts*.

Printed in the United States of America.

Contributors

CONSULTING EDITOR

LEE A. FLEISHER, MD, FACC, FAHA
Robert D. Dripps Professor and Chair of Anesthesiology and Critical Care, Professor of Medicine, Perelman School of Medicine, University of Pennsylvania, Philadelphia, Pennsylvania, USA

EDITOR

ALEXANDER A. HANNENBERG, MD
Ariadne Labs, Harvard T.H. Chan School of Public Health, Brigham and Women's Hospital, Tufts University School of Medicine, Boston, Massachusetts, USA

AUTHORS

JOSEPH F. ANSWINE, MD, FASA
Partner, Riverside Anesthesia Associates, Staff Anesthesiologist, University of Pittsburgh Medical Center (UPMC) Pinnacle, Harrisburg, Pennsylvania, USA; Clinical Associate Professor, Department of Anesthesiology and Perioperative Medicine, Pennsylvania State University Hospital, Hershey, Pennsylvania, USA; Staff Anesthesiologist, Geisinger Health System, Danville, Pennsylvania, USA

ALEXANDER F. ARRIAGA, MD, MPH, ScD
Department of Anesthesiology, Perioperative and Pain Medicine, Brigham and Women's Hospital, Ariadne Labs, Center for Surgery and Public Health, Boston, Massachusetts, USA

CARLOS A. ARTIME, MD
Associate Professor, Vice Chair of Finance and Operations, Department of Anesthesiology, McGovern Medical School, The University of Texas Health Science Center at Houston, Houston, Texas, USA

JOSHUA A. BLOOMSTONE, MD, MSc, FASA
Senior Vice President for Clinical Innovation, Associate Medical Director, Envision Center for Quality and Patient Safety, Envision Physician Services, Plantation, Florida, USA; Clinical Professor of Anesthesiology, The University of Arizona College of Medicine-Phoenix, Phoenix, Arizona, USA; Honorary Associate Professor, Division of Surgery and Interventional Sciences, University College London, Centre for Perioperative Medicine, London, England

RICHARD BOTNEY, MD
Assistant Professor, Staff Anesthesiologist, Department of Anesthesiology and Perioperative Medicine, Oregon Health & Science University, Portland, Oregon, USA

AMANDA R. BURDEN, MD
Professor of Anesthesiology, Director, Clinical Skills and Simulation, Vice Chair and Chief of Faculty Affairs, Cooper Medical School of Rowan University, Cooper University Healthcare, CMSRU Simulation Center, Camden, New Jersey, USA

BARBARA K. BURIAN, PhD
Senior Research Psychologist, NASA Ames Research Center, Moffett Field, California, USA

CHARLES E. COWLES Jr, MD, MBA, FASA
Associate Professor, Chief Safety Officer, Department of Anesthesiology and Perioperative Medicine, The University of Texas MD Anderson Cancer Center, Houston, Texas, USA

MEGAN DELISLE, MD, MPH, MSc
Department of Surgery, University of Manitoba, Winnipeg, Manitoba, Canada

R. KEY DISMUKES, PhD
NASA Chief Scientist for Aerospace Human Factors (Retired), Moffett Field, California, USA

BRENDA A. GENTZ, MD
Associate Professor of Anesthesiology, University of Arizona College of Medicine-Tucson, Banner - University Medical Center Tucson, Tucson, Arizona, USA

CARIN A. HAGBERG, MD
Chief Academic Officer, Division Head, Anesthesiology, Critical Care and Pain Medicine, Bud Johnson Clinical Distinguished Chair, Department of Anesthesiology and Perioperative Medicine, The University of Texas MD Anderson Cancer Center, Houston, Texas, USA

ALEXANDER A. HANNENBERG, MD
Ariadne Labs, Harvard T.H. Chan School of Public Health, Brigham and Women's Hospital, Tufts University School of Medicine, Boston, Massachusetts, USA

JOY L. HAWKINS, MD
Professor of Anesthesiology, Director of Obstetric Anesthesia, University of Colorado School of Medicine, Aurora, Colorado, USA

BENJAMIN T. HOUSEMAN, MD, PhD, FASA
Director, Memorial Healthcare System Anesthesiology Residency Program, Anesthesiologist, Envision Physician Services, Pembroke Pines, Florida, USA

SACHIN KHETERPAL, MD, MBA
Department of Anesthesiology, University of Michigan, Ann Arbor, Michigan, USA

THOMAS T. KLUMPNER, MD
Departments of Anesthesiology and Obstetrics and Gynecology, University of Michigan, Ann Arbor, Michigan, USA

GERALD MACCIOLI, MD, MBA, FCCM, FASA
Advisor to the Board, Quick'r Care, Miami, Florida, USA

NADER N. MASSARWEH, MD, MPH
Center for Innovations in Quality, Effectiveness and Safety, Michael E. DeBakey VA Medical Center, Michael E. DeBakey Department of Surgery, Baylor College of Medicine,

Section of Health Services Research, Department of Medicine, Baylor College of Medicine, Houston, Texas, USA

JOSEPH MCISAAC, MD, MS, MBA, CPE, FASA
Clinical Professor of Anesthesiology, University of Connecticut School of Medicine, Farmington, Connecticut, USA; Supervisory Medical Officer, National Disaster Medical System, US Department of Health and Human Services, Washington, DC, USA

MARK E. NUNNALLY, MD
Professor, Departments of Anesthesiology, Perioperative Care and Pain Medicine, Neurology, Surgery and Medicine, Director, Adult Critical Care Services, NYU Langone Health, NYU Langone Medical Center, New York, New York, USA

ARPIT PATEL, MD
Assistant Professor, Department of Anesthesiology, Perioperative Care and Pain Medicine, NYU Langone Health, NYU Langone Medical Center, New York, New York, USA

MAY C.M. PIAN-SMITH, MD, MS
Center for Medical Simulation, Department of Anesthesia, Critical Care and Pain Medicine, Massachusetts General Hospital, Boston, Massachusetts, USA

PAUL POTNURU, MD
Assistant Professor, Department of Anesthesiology, McGovern Medical School, The University of Texas Health Science Center at Houston, Houston, Texas, USA

DEMIAN SZYLD, MD, EdM
Department of Emergency Medicine, Brigham and Women's Hospital, Center for Medical Simulation, Boston, Massachusetts, USA

Contents

Many factors come together probabilistically to affect clinician response to critical events in the operating room; no 2 critical events are alike. These factors involve 4 primary domains: (1) the event itself, (2) the individual anesthetist(s), (3) the operating room team, and (4) the resources available and environments in which the event occurs. Appreciating these factors, anticipating how they create vulnerabilities for error and poor response, and actively addressing those vulnerabilities (before events occur as well as during) will help clinicians manage critical event response more effectively and avoid errors.

This article explores high-fidelity simulation in anesthesiology education and provides strategies for its use to improve management of critical events. Educational theories that underlie the use of simulation are described. High-fidelity simulation is useful in teaching technical (diagnostic and procedural) and nontechnical (communication and professionalism) skills, including crisis resource management (CRM) skills. The practice of CRM is fundamental to ensuring patient safety during critical events and to the safe practice of anesthesiology, and its critical elements are presented. A discussion of the use of high-fidelity simulation to learn to combine highly complex procedural skills and CRM is also provided.

Simulation-based education improves health care professionals' performance in managing critical events. Limitations to widespread uptake of high-fidelity simulation include barriers related to training, technology, and time. Alternatives to high-fidelity simulation that overcome these barriers include in situ simulation, classroom-based simulation, telesimulation, observed simulation, screen-based simulation, and game-based simulation. Some settings have limited access to onsite expert facilitation to design, implement, and guide participants through simulation-based education. Alternatives to onsite expert debriefing in these settings include teledebriefing, scripted debriefing, and within-group debriefing. A combination of these alternatives promotes successful implementation and maintenance of simulation-based education for managing critical health care events.

Postoperative complications, which occur in approximately 23% of surgeries, are a major source of patient mortality. Some of these deaths may be preventable. This article explores factors and contexts during the intraoperative period, in the postanesthesia care unit, perioperatively, and after discharge that may represent opportunities to intervene and prevent mortality after a potentially treatable complication. Tools to improve the identification and response to life-threatening complications in these unique care settings are discussed.

Critical events are rare and stressful. These properties make reliance on memory for clinical management highly susceptible to failure. In the past 10 to 20 years, health care has begun to accept the experience of aviation and other high-reliability organizations in addressing failure to rescue from these events through a combination of practice through simulation and the introduction of cognitive aids, known as checklists or emergency manuals. Cognitive aids have a persuasive body of evidence from simulation studies to establish their value in improving clinician performance. However, their introduction to practice is more complex than distribution of the tools.

Debriefing after perioperative crises (eg, cardiac arrest, massive hemorrhage) is a well-described practice that can provide benefits to individuals, teams, and health systems. Debriefing has also been embraced by high-stakes industries outside of health care. Yet, in studies of actual clinical practice, there are many critical events that do not get debriefed. This article explores the gap that exists between principle and reality and the factors and strategies to offer opportunities to reflect on actual critical events, when indicated, across the increasing scope of environments where anesthesia care is provided.

There are many forms of mass casualty events, including mass trauma, exposure to radiation and chemical agents, biological exposure (pandemics and bioterrorism), or a combination of insults. The underlying theme is that the number and severity of patients outstrip the resources available. These events are more common than thought. Planning and preparation allow institutions to better respond to the patient surge and thus mitigate the consequences—ultimately saving lives and reducing morbidity.

Obstetric Hemorrhage

Joy L. Hawkins

Peripartum hemorrhage is a leading cause of maternal morbidity and mortality. Anesthesiologists must be familiar with conditions associated with hemorrhage that are unique to labor and delivery and not seen elsewhere in their practice. Regardless of etiology, early recognition and timely treatment of obstetric hemorrhage is necessary to prevent significant blood loss. Massive transfusion protocols are crucial to successful resuscitation, and providers should also consider use of cell salvage, uterine artery embolization, and anti-fibrinolytics. Because more than half the deaths due to hemorrhage are preventable, multidisciplinary care bundles should be used on every labor and delivery unit.

Intraoperative Cardiac Arrest

Benjamin T. Houseman, Joshua A. Bloomstone, and Gerald Maccioli

Cardiac arrest in the operating room and in the immediate postoperative period is a potentially catastrophic event that is almost always witnessed and is frequently anticipated. Perioperative crises and perioperative cardiac arrest, although often catastrophic, are frequently managed in a timely and directed manner because practitioners have a deep knowledge of the patient's medical condition and details of recent procedures. It is hoped that the approaches described here, along with approaches for the rapid identification and management of specific high-stakes clinical scenarios, will help anesthesiologists continue to improve patient outcomes.

The Lost Airway

Paul Potnuru, Carlos A. Artime, and Carin A. Hagberg

Management of the unanticipated difficult airway is one of the most relevant and challenging crisis management scenarios encountered in clinical anesthesia practice. Several guidelines and approaches have been developed to assist clinicians in navigating this high-acuity scenario. In the most serious cases, the clinician may encounter a failed airway that results from failure to ventilate an anesthetized patient via facemask or supraglottic airway or intubate the patient with an endotracheal tube. This dreaded cannot intubate, cannot oxygenate situation necessitates emergency invasive access. This article reviews the incidence, management, and complications of the failed airway and training issues related to its management.

The Septic Patient

Arpit Patel and Mark E. Nunnally

Anesthesiologists are uniquely positioned to facilitate emergent care of patients with sepsis in the perioperative setting. A subset of sepsis patients presents with surgical pathology. Emphasis is on timely intervention with source control, antibiotic therapy, and aggressive resuscitation. Ileus, aspiration, and cardiovascular collapse must be considered when inducing patients with sepsis. Dynamic fluid responsiveness may prove an effective tool in minimizing over-resuscitation. Assessment of circulatory failure and drug therapy involves an understanding of preload, afterload, and contractility. Timely, targeted resuscitation and early source control have persisted and remain fundamental to sepsis care.

Oxygen supply failures are potentially life-threatening and are often associated with death or brain damage. Knowledge of how oxygen is supplied is essential for understanding how failures are caused and their management. Even though safety mechanisms exist to reduce the likelihood of a supply failure, events still occur. Simulation studies have identified knowledge and performance gaps in management of supply failures. A straightforward approach to immediate management of these critical events is provided.

ANESTHESIOLOGY CLINICS

FORTHCOMING ISSUES

March 2021
Neuroanesthesia
Jeffrey Kirsch and Cindy Lien, *Editors*

June 2021
Enhanced Recovery after Surgery and
Perioperative Medicine
Michael Scott, Anton Krige, and Michael
Grocott, *Editors*

RECENT ISSUES

September 2020
Pediatric Anesthesia
Alison Perate and Vanessa Olbrecht,
Editors

June 2020
Gender, Racial, and Socioeconomic Issues in
Perioperative Medicine
Katherine Forkin, Lauren Dunn, and
Edward Nemergut, *Editors*

SERIES OF RELATED INTEREST

Pediatric Clinics

THE CLINICS ARE AVAILABLE ONLINE!
Access your subscription at:
www.theclinics.com

Foreword

The Actions That Define Us: Our Response to Critical Events

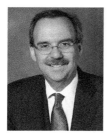

Lee A. Fleisher, MD, FACC, FAHA
Consulting Editor

As anesthesiologists, we are used to hearing that our job is 99% boredom and 1% sheer terror. While many of us believe that this description is far from accurate, our ability to "rescue" a patient who is having a complication and recovery and learn after a critical event is paramount. The method by which we learn to address such events is continuing to evolve as our knowledge of human cognitive traps grows. In this issue of *Anesthesiology Clinics*, experts in the field describe some of these general concepts and approaches. This is further enhanced by articles addressing specific events by true experts in their respective fields.

In deciding who could assemble a group of experts and provide a vision for this issue, one name came to mind. Alexander Hannenberg, MD has been a leader in our specialty for decades. I personally met Alex while he was leading the American Society of Anesthesiologists (ASA) efforts in quality and quality measurement for the AMA Physician Consortium for Performance Improvement. He served as president of the ASA and as its Chief Quality Officer. He is now Clinical Professor of Anesthesiology at Tufts University School of Medicine and is a faculty member in the Safe Surgery Program at Ariadne Labs. He has given much of his time as a founding board member to the important Lifebox USA. He has assembled an amazing group of authors to teach us how to learn and do the best for our patients every day.

Lee A. Fleisher, MD, FACC, FAHA
3400 Spruce Street
Dulles 680
Philadelphia, PA 19104, USA

E-mail address:
Lee.Fleisher@uphs.upenn.edu

Anesthesiology Clin 38 (2020) xiii
https://doi.org/10.1016/j.anclin.2020.09.002
1932-2275/20/© 2020 Published by Elsevier Inc.

Preface

"When Our Patients Need Us Most"

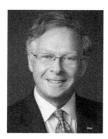

Alexander A. Hannenberg, MD
Editor

The contents of this issue of *Anesthesiology Clinics* are the stuff of which anesthesiologist nightmares are made. The clinical events addressed here share 2 key features: they are uncommon and they are serious. No single clinician will reliably have recent experience in managing these events, and avoiding significant patient harm from the event depends on expert management.

These features, along with their unpredictable occurrence, make study of the clinical management much less amenable to research tools, such as randomized controlled study. Simulation-based research plays an outsized role in the body of knowledge on effective strategies in critical event management. Similarly, simulation training is a core component of preparedness. We include 2 articles on different approaches to simulation training.

Much of the clinical guidance provided in these articles is available to us from observation, debriefing, and qualitative study of the uncommon events addressed here. For example, the article on Mass Casualty by McIsaac and Gentz draws from the lessons learned from numerous catastrophic events around the world over a period of decades. The multiple dimensions in which debriefing of real events can improve care, including system strengthening, are described by Arriaga and colleagues. The risks of these events not only to the patient, but also to the "second victim," emerge in their discussion.

The issue is organized into 2 sections. In the first, topics of importance to improving management of critical events in general are discussed. Behavioral psychology, simulation, predictive tools, cognitive aids, and debriefing are addressed. The second section addresses a handful of specific uncommon, high-stakes clinical scenarios. The authors of those articles repeatedly point back to the cross-cutting topics to provide context for the management guidance they provide.

Anesthesiology Clin 38 (2020) xv–xvi
https://doi.org/10.1016/j.anclin.2020.09.001
1932-2275/20/© 2020 Published by Elsevier Inc.

anesthesiology.theclinics.com

The authors have included scores of recommended practices throughout the issue. As you prioritize these for your practice, bear in mind the essential need for a deliberate implementation strategy to move the improvements from bookshelf to bedside. As entrepreneur Guy Kawasaki has said, "ideas are easy, implementation is hard."[1] I'm not sure about the first part, but the second part is very true and makes or breaks improvement efforts every day.

Ghaferi and colleagues make the point that what distinguishes good hospitals from bad ones is their capacity to rescue from complications, much more so than the frequency with which complications occur.[2] Though we have included a specific article focused on rescue, in an important way this is the theme of the entire issue.

I feel fortunate to have engaged such a highly qualified and prominent group of authors for this issue. The fact that they were writing and editing in the midst of a global pandemic challenging anesthesia departments around the world makes their contributions even more remarkable and my gratitude even greater.

Together, we hope that the content of this issue will extinguish some of our recurring nightmares and improve the care of our patients when they need us most.

Alexander A. Hannenberg, MD
Ariadne Labs
401 Park Drive 3-West
Boston, MA 02215, USA

E-mail address:
ahannenberg@ariadnelabs.org

REFERENCES

1. Kawasaki G. Ideas are easy, implementation is hard. Forbes, November 2004;4. Available at: https://www.forbes.com/2004/11/04/cx_gk_1104artofthestart/#31ec326a1cc5. Accessed September 7, 2020.
2. Ghaferi AA, Birkmeyer JD, Dimick JB. Complications, failure to rescue, and mortality with major inpatient surgery in Medicare patients. Ann Surg 2009;250(6): 1029–34. https://doi.org/10.1097/sla.0b013e3181bef697.

Why We Fail to Rescue During Critical Events

Barbara K. Burian, PhD*, R. Key Dismukes, PhD

KEYWORDS

- Critical event • System 1 & 2 thinking • Cognitive bias • Working memory • Fatigue
- Crew resource management • Cognitive aids

KEY POINTS

- Critical event response in the operating room (OR) is affected by the probabilistic combination of factors involving the event itself, the individuals involved and their interactions as a team, and the available resources and environments in which the event occurs.
- Different events pose different challenges and even the same type of event may evolve in different ways. Their complexity, time-criticality, and degree to which symptoms match event prototypical diagnostic criteria, as well as patient demographics and comorbidities, all have possible effects.
- The challenges for individual clinicians responding effectively to critical events are primarily cognitive in nature (eg, overloaded working memory, distractions, cognitive biases leading to missed cues and misdiagnoses, and novel events requiring more focused and effortful system 2 thinking), although personal factors, such as fatigue and chronic stress, also can have real effects.
- The ways that individuals in the OR do or do not come together as a coherent team greatly affects critical event response. How clinicians apply the principles of crew resource management—leadership and followership, team communication and coordination, situation awareness, and shared mental models—substantially affect team effectiveness.
- Obviously, the equipment, materials, and other resources available (including fellow humans) as well as the environments in which the event occurs can have a great impact on critical event response. Several environment types have an influence, ranging from the physical and work environment to the institutional cultural, community, and certification and regulatory environments.

Funding and Conflicts of Interest: Neither author received funding related to this work other than Dr B.K. Burian's salary from NASA; neither author reports any commercial interests or conflicts of interest.
NASA Ames Research Center, Building N262, Room H101, Mail Stop 262-4, Moffett Field, CA 94035-1000, USA
* Corresponding author.
E-mail address: Barbara.K.Burian@nasa.gov

Anesthesiology Clin 38 (2020) 727–743
https://doi.org/10.1016/j.anclin.2020.08.009   **anesthesiology.theclinics.com**
1932-2275/20/© 2020 National Aeronautics and Space Administration. Published by Elsevier Inc.

INTRODUCTION

The patient was a 55-year-old, 75-kg woman with a prior inferior myocardial infarction (MI) and breast cancer, to undergo reconstructive breast (left) surgery after a complete mastectomy. The procedure was delayed for more than 4 hours because of operating room (OR) scheduling problems and staff availability. The surgical resident was extremely anxious to begin and the anesthesiology attending had not had an expected break for lunch 2 hours earlier. Anesthesia was induced without problem and the patient was prepped and draped. Just prior to incision, the patient's heart rate suddenly began to drop (**Fig. 1**).

The first year clinical anesthesia resident (CA1) increased the patient's oxygen to 100% and administered 0.2-mg atropine. A nurse summoned the anesthesiology attending STAT. A minute later the attending arrived and administered 10-μg epinephrine as the heart rate continued to drop. The surgical resident complained about the delay as the anesthesia attending instructed the CA1 to perform chest compressions while he administered an arrest dose of epinephrine, asked the OR nurse to call for help, and started to set up an epinephrine infusion. The very short CA1 complied but even standing on her tiptoes had trouble administering compressions at an adequate depth. The surgical attending kept entering and exiting the OR asking about progress. The anesthesiologist first inadvertently programmed the epinephrine infusion at 1500 μg/min (the maximum dosing for dopamine) and then immediately corrected to 10 μg/min. A circulating nurse, on his own volition, went and obtained a crash cart; the anesthesiologist was unaware that it was available as he worked frantically to address the patient's increasing bradycardia and switch with the CA1 in providing compressions.

The surgical resident continued to ask how much longer it would be until the patient was stabilized. While doing chest compressions, the anesthesiology attending noticed that the anesthetic gas was still on and he immediately told the CA1 to turn it off. He then told the surgical resident that they needed to focus on stabilizing the patient and postpone the reconstructive surgery.

As illustrated in this scenario (and analyzed later), how anesthetists respond to a critical event is driven by factors in 4 broad, interrelated domains:

1. The event itself
2. The individual anesthetist(s) involved
3. The OR team
4. Available resources and the environment in which the event occurs

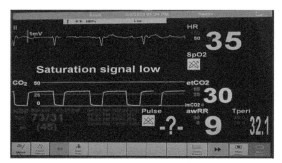

Fig. 1. Severe bradycardia. (*From* SafeSurg2015. OR Emergency with OR Crisis Checklist. Available at: https://www.youtube.com/watch?v=iaHiSYR11u0&feature=youtu.be.)

Human factors experts no longer talk about "human error" as an isolated phenomenon; instead, we talk about characteristics of an entire system that can increase or decrease the probability of errors or having difficulty in responding to critical events.

Some of the primary factors in each of these 4 areas are reviewed (**Fig. 2**) and then how they can come together, probabilistically, to bear on critical event response. General observations and recommendations about ways to change systems to increase effective responses to critical events are made throughout.

THE EVENT

The characteristics of critical events may vary along several closely related dimensions.[1] In medicine, the first dimension pertains to **how it evolves over time:** Is its occurrence sudden and abrupt or slow and insidious? How obvious and clear-cut are the cues and symptoms that let the anesthesiologist and other clinicians know that something is amiss? Conditions with a sudden onset and/or with cues and symptoms that obviously are abnormal and are alerted generally are identified and addressed more quickly than those whose abnormal cues and symptoms are insidious and slower to evolve.[2]

The second dimension involves the degree to which cues and symptoms match the clinician's mental model or understanding of what cues and symptoms of that

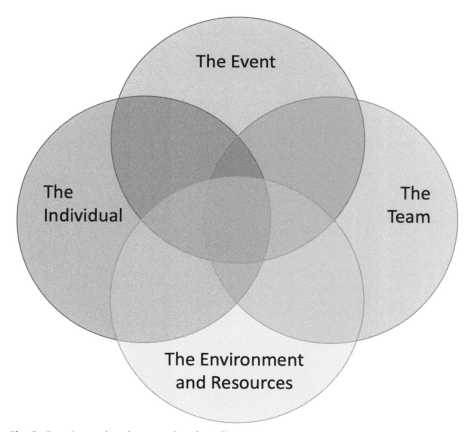

Fig. 2. Four interrelated areas related to clinician response to critical events.

particular condition should look like. In other words, how closely do they **match known diagnostic criteria** for that type of event? Clinicians, like other professionals, are faster to respond and are more likely to diagnose a condition correctly when the symptoms and cues closely match those of a prototypical condition. When the symptoms observed are common to several kinds of critical events, however, full event response may be slowed because clinicians must perform a differential diagnosis to ensure correct and complete treatment.

The third dimension involves the **complexity of the event** and the associated demands of the required response. Event complexity and demands encompass not only the type of event but also how severe it is and underlying patient comorbidities that affect treatment. A teenager's mild anaphylactic drug reaction is less demanding and complex than malignant hyperthermia in a 67-year-old patient with a pacemaker and coronary artery disease.

The fourth primary dimension is event **time criticality:** How quickly must clinicians act to save the patient and keep him/her from harm? With increased time pressure come increased stress and workload and a greater likelihood of clinicians making a mistake.[3]

THE INDIVIDUAL

How individual clinicians respond to critical events is driven predominantly by the fundamental nature of human cognition and cognitive processing, although there also are factors associated with the specific person, such as personality, level of training and knowledge, and variable factors, such as hunger, fatigue, and physical health.

Cognition

Why do skilled and conscientious experts, such as anesthesiologists, sometimes have difficulty responding correctly to critical events? For years it has been assumed that, if an expert made consequential errors, something was wrong with the expert—they lacked skill or were careless. But now there is an enormous amount of research showing that in most cases the issue is not deficiency on the part of the individual but rather the fundamental nature of the cognitive processes and how those processes operate in challenging situations.[4,5]

In responding to a critical event, anesthetists must first be aware (through sensation and perception) that something is wrong and must selectively focus attention on relevant cues and information, hold this information in working memory, and combine it with previously learned information stored in long-term memory to determine what is going on and what to do about it. Each cognitive process holds special challenges for critical event response (**Table 1**). What the anesthetist does with all that information in working memory is influenced by (1) how 2 fundamental modes of cognitive processing operate, (2) cognitive biases and heuristics, (3) interruptions and distractions, and (4) levels of fatigue and acute stress.

Different modes of information processing

There are 2 modes or systems with which the human brain/mind processes information[6] and both play central roles in critical event response. System 1 operates automatically outside of direct conscious control, drawing on the enormous amount of information stored in associative memory to recognize and interpret situations quickly and respond appropriately. System 1 capabilities are acquired throughout life, some quite naturally, such as learning a language; others develop over a lifetime of experience in specific domains, such as medicine. In critical events, it is system 1 thinking

Table 1
Introduction to human cognition 101 (and related challenges for critical event response)

Basic Cognition	Challenge for Critical Event Response
Sensation and perception: taking in information from our surroundings, typically through our sensory systems (visual, auditory, olfactory, tactile, proprioception, etc.) and organizing, interpreting, and making sense of it	• Too many stimuli can make it difficult to focus on that which is relevant and to recall learned information and think about what should be done. ■ *Recommendation*: turn OFF music and eliminate nonessential and nonpertinent communication.
Attention: selective focus and concentration on specific perceived stimuli or information while ignoring other stimuli and information	• What we do and do not pay attention to during a critical event can be adversely affected by cognitive biases and inappropriately applied heuristics; this can lead to misdiagnosis of the problem (see below). ■ *Recommendation*: deliberately pause from time to time, step back mentally and check your assumptions. • Attention is like a spotlight —we can pay attention to only a few things at any one time and it is easy to fixate on just 1 or 2. ■ *Recommendation*: adjust, back-and-forth, the width of your attention spotlight between narrow band (focusing on just a few things) to wide band (assessing the status of the overall situation). ■ *Recommendation*: when in narrow-band mode, shift your attention around so that you do not miss relevant information or cues and ask others, "What am I missing?"
Long-term memory: a vast cognitive storage system where memories and learned information are encoded and stored, relatively permanently, for later retrieval and use	• Our ability to recall learned information is often impaired when under stress and time pressure. ■ *Recommendation*: refresh your memory of critical events and appropriate treatments before you encounter them in real life by staying current on the literature and seeking out training activities. ■ *Recommendation*: use critical event checklists and cognitive aids during event response and use them as study aids other times.

(continued on next page)

Table 1 *(continued)*	
Basic Cognition	**Challenge for Critical Event Response**
Working memory: a temporary short-term memory system in which perceived information and/or information retrieved from long-term memory are held, computed, manipulated, evaluated, and used in cognitive processes, such as decision-making	• The amount of information we can hold in working memory and how long we can retain it is severely limited (even on a good day) and both shrink when under stress. ▪ *Recommendation*: make written notes or ask someone to write down critical information (eg, times events occurred, drugs/doses administered and when) and ask others to check your calculations.
Prospective memory: remembering to complete a deferred action at a later time when it is relevant or appropriate	• Prospective memory is inherently quite vulnerable to forgetting, especially under the high workload, interruptions, and distractions common in critical events. ▪ *Recommendation*: use devices (eg, timer on cell phone), create explicit intentions and cues, and ask others to help you remember to complete tasks that must be delayed until later.

that allows responding automatically to things, such as a disconnected anesthesia circuit, without deliberate mentation. Much of the work of experienced professionals depends heavily on system 1 to quickly recognize and respond to a vast range of situations.

System 2 is associated with effortful mentation required when making complex calculations, dealing with novel situations, and making difficult choices. In contrast with system 1, which is fast and has virtually unlimited capacity, system 2 is slow and narrow-band; only 1 thing can be focused on at a time. System 2 depends heavily on the executive processes of focal attention and working memory. (Other terms with different emphases sometimes are used for these 2 modes of processing, for example, automatic processing and controlled processing.)[7]

The 2 systems work together; both control attention. System 1 automatically orients attention to what experience has found to be the critical aspects of the current situation, but system 2 enables deliberately redirecting attention—especially in uncertain situations—and counteracting the heuristic errors and cognitive biases in system 1 thinking that can cause missing important information or leading in the wrong direction.

Cognitive biases and heuristics

As clinicians develop experience, they develop mental short-cuts (heuristics) to quicken the diagnostic process.[8] Many heuristics involve automatically recognizing a familiar pattern and the underlying cause. Because they operate automatically, heuristics are fast and efficient. The volume of clinical work would be impossible to accomplish if relying solely on slower system 2 thinking. Heuristics generally take us in the right direction, but because they work with incomplete information, they sometimes mislead. Additionally, various cognitive biases unconsciously distort recognition of situations.[8,9] For example, everyone is subject to confirmation bias, which favors information supporting initial diagnosis and neglects disconfirmatory evidence. **Table 2** provides examples of common biases and heuristic errors that can lead clinicians astray in all situations but especially in time-pressured critical events.

Recommendation: Groopman[11] suggests that when making diagnoses, clinicians periodically step back and ask, "Is there anything that does not fit this diagnosis?" and "What else could it be?" to try bring any cognitive biases to conscious awareness. This can be difficult to do in time-pressured critical events, but is even more important then.

Interruptions and distractions

Interruptions and distractions, particularly during critical events, often are unavoidable.[12] A task is begun and someone asks a question, arrives with needed units of pack red blood cells or the crash cart, or we interrupt ourselves by diverting our attention to some other task that seems more critical. When interrupted or distracted, we are vulnerable to forgetting to resume the interrupted task and to forgetting where we left off within the task[13]—did I already give a third dose of amiodarone to my patient in cardiac arrest or not? When interruptions and distractions are frequent, the limited capacity of attention and working memory can be overwhelmed, undercutting the ability to manage tasks systematically and making clinicians more vulnerable to forgetting to perform intended actions[12] (see **Table 1**).

High workload, interruptions, and distractions can also make clinicians more vulnerable to habit capture in that we forget our intention to deviate from or modify a normal, habitual procedure in a particular case. Under challenging work conditions, system 1 tends to respond automatically to familiar situations in the habitual manner, unless monitored and over-ruled by system 2.

Table 2 Common heuristic errors and cognitive biases in medicine	
Heuristic Error or Cognitive Bias	**Description**
Strong but wrong	Usually the heuristic is correct but not in this situation.
Just wrong	A heuristic that works in another, dissimilar, situation is applied incorrectly in this situation.
Availability bias	Recently seen or discussed diagnoses or situations influence clinicians to see it again now, with a new patient.
Confirmation bias	Looking for/seeing evidence that supports assumptions and ignoring/not looking for evidence that does not
Attribution error	Unduly forming a diagnosis and/or opinion about someone based on their race, age, gender, appearance, etc.
Anchoring	Being overly influenced by the first available information when formulating a diagnosis
Premature closure	The tendency to settle on the first diagnosis thought of early in the diagnostic process and to not consider others
Commission bias	The impulse and need to "do something" rather than just "stand there"

Data from Refs.[10,11]

Recommendation: be thoughtful about when you do and do not let others interrupt and distract you. During a difficult intubation, when someone asks an unrelated question, tell them to "Standby" or say, "In a minute," so you can focus on the task at hand.[3,12]

Recommendation: make notes (eg, put sticky notes on a monitor) or get others involved in helping you remember that you need to perform an action in an atypical way or that some actions normally performed should not be. Best of all, create a physical barrier to performing the normal action (may not be feasible during a rushed critical event but could be during normal situations). For example, put a band of tape across the bin in the Omnicell™ drawer holding a drug you would habitually use but is contraindicated in this specific case.

Note that 2 challenges in using on-the-fly physical barriers are (1) you have to pick one that cannot be defeated automatically, without thinking, and (2) you have to remember to remove it after case completion so it does not affect actions in later cases.

Critical event response, however, often requires interleaving multiple tasks; clinicians must interrupt themselves as they shift their attention from one thing to another and back again. (This mistakenly is referred to as multitasking; humans usually are not truly performing several tasks simultaneously but instead shifting back and forth among them.[14])

Recommendation: be as intentional as possible with how you interrupt your actions on one task and shift your attention to another. Make a mental note of where you are leaving off and what you will do next on that task when you return to it.[13] If possible, make written notes or elicit help from others in remembering.

One of the risks faced when shifting among tasks is becoming fixated on 1 challenging task and forgetting to shift attention back to the others.[15]

Recommendation: try to regularly find time to mentally step back from what you are doing, not only to review the overall status of the situation but also to remind yourself of what you might be forgetting to do.

Levels of fatigue and acute stress

It is well understood that fatigue has a negative effect on human performance, including that of doctors.[16,17] Caffeine, splashing cold water on one's face, or taking a short break may help briefly but typically are not practical during critical event response, and fatigue can delay awareness that such an event is even happening. The psychophysiologic arousal common with critical events[2] may help overcome some fatigue effects initially but only up to a point; high levels of arousal associated with stressful situations—particularly when tasks may be challenging—have a negative effect on human performance and cognitive processing (see **Table 1**).

Acute stress occurs when workload and task complexity threaten to overload the limited capacity of a clinician's attention and working memory. This generates anxiety, which in turn disrupts effective management of attention, undercutting situation assessment, management of competing task demands, and effective communication, among other errors.[3]

Recommendation: when fatigued or stressed, get help: get others involved in helping to perform and remember tasks and actions, provide second opinions, and check your work.

Additionally, research suggests that repeated exposure to simulated critical events may help reduce stress effects of real events when they occur.[18]

Recommendation: regularly participate in critical event simulation training.[19]

Personal Factors

Of course, various personal factors also mediate how clinicians respond during critical events. Some are enduring, trait characteristics (with minimal modifiability once achieving "expert in a domain" status), such as personality, knowledge, skills, abilities, and level of training. Others are state characteristics—such as hunger, fatigue, physical and mental health, chronic stress (eg, seriously ill family member), and length of time since relevant training—that fluctuate over the course of minutes, days, or months.

How each factor comes together and interacts with the others and the effects they have during critical events vary greatly. Furthermore, some have greater bearing than others on clinician response; a moderately tired anesthesia attending with 12-years of experience likely always performs better than a well-rested CA2.

THE TEAM

Several major airline accidents occurred in the 1970s in which competent flight crews crashed aircraft with no mechanical problems because they did not draw on all potentially available information and communicate effectively (**Fig. 3**A). This led airlines, military flight organizations, and NASA to develop crew resource management (CRM) programs (**Fig. 3**B). One tenet of CRM encourages all team members to share their understanding of situations, so that they are all working from the same page (ie, ensure shared situation awareness).[20] In particular, subordinate team members are encouraged to be assertive (respectfully) when they see problems not being addressed. CRM also emphasizes leadership, encouraging subordinates to communicate, situation awareness, coordination, problem-solving, and decision-making.

CRM has been adopted in medicine, to some extent, and has been found to improve team performance.[21–23] When there is an identified leader who effectively elicits and structures the help of others, and when all team members effectively communicate with each other, team situational awareness, shared mental models, informed decision-making, and effective critical event response tend to naturally follow (**Box 1**).

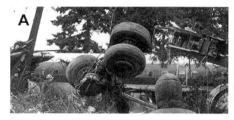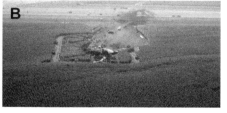

Fig. 3. (*A*) United Airlines Flight 173 accident, December 28, 1978, Portland, Oregon. The aircraft crashed due to fuel exhaustion while crew's attention was focused on a landing gear problem. Ten people were killed and 34 were injured out of 189 people on board. (*B*). United Airlines Flight 232 accident, July 19, 1989, Sioux City, Iowa. The aircraft experienced a complete failure of all 3 hydraulics systems and completed an emergency landing using differential thrust. Of the 11 crew and 285 passengers on board, 111 perished. This type of failure was thought to be impossible (and not survivable); the survival of 185 people is credited, in large part, to the excellent CRM of the crew. (*From* Loss of Thrust in Both Engines After Encountering a Flock of Birds and Subsequent Ditching on the Hudson River US Airways Flight 1549 Airbus A320-214, N106US Weehawken, New Jersey January 15, 2009.)

> **Box 1**
> **Crew resource management**
>
> Leadership—a leader is clearly identified and that leader elicits help (when needed) and establishes the roles of others on the team. The leader actively solicits information and suggestions from others, monitors the status of the overall situation, and ensures that all available resources are used.
>
> Followership—others in the original OR team, and any others asked to help, follow the guidance and direction of the leader, complete assigned actions, and offer observations and suggestions at appropriate times.
>
> Team communication—respectful but direct, relevant, timely, and well-timed information sharing among all team members.
>
> Team coordination—synchronized and timely performance of actions by all members of the team. Possible need for equipment and resources not immediately available is predicted and timely actions are taken to obtain it.
>
> Team situational awareness—the joint and common understanding among all team members about the current status of a situation and how it might naturally progress on its current trajectory.
>
> Shared mental models—the joint and common understanding about the nature of a situation (diagnosis, etiology, and so forth), what should be done about it (if anything), and who should be doing it and when.

CRM applies to normal situations as well as critical events. A version of CRM has been coined "Crisis Resource Management" by Fanning and colleagues,[24] which includes not only aspects of traditional CRM (eg, designate leadership, communicate effectively, use all available information, and mobilize resources) but also additional components to help structure and guide team critical event response (eg, call for help early, know the environment, and use cognitive aids).

THE ENVIRONMENT AND AVAILABLE RESOURCES

Five primary environments can affect how critical events are managed.

1. The physical environment where the event occurs: an OR, intensive care unit, emergency room, or a field outside, near the site of a mass casualty situation
2. The work environment: are practices and workflow within the institution (in particular, the site where the event occurs) orderly and logical or disorganized and chaotic? Is the facility affiliated with a large academic university or is it an inner-city trauma 1 hospital, a medium-sized or small community hospital, a rural and remote clinic, or something else? Each comes with different resources in the number of personnel and their clinical specialties and the cognitive aids and equipment and supplies available which, in turn, affect the demands on and support for clinicians who are directly responding to a critical event.
3. The institution's cultural environment: does the facility have open, supportive relationships among people and across disciplines or is it strictly hierarchical, rigid, and closed? Is it a learning institution with a just culture ethos in which mistakes and problems are seen as opportunities to improve or is it a culture imbued with suspicion and oriented toward blame (**Box 2**)?
4. The larger community and national environment[25]
5. The certification and regulatory environment: these affect the institution and individuals practicing there and can have subtle (or sometimes, not so subtle) effects on critical event management.

Box 2
Safety management systems concepts

Learning institution: an organization that consistently and systematically collects, monitors, and analyzes data regarding patient safety, practices and workflow, and quality improvement initiatives and uses those findings to implement changes and new improvement initiatives.

Just culture: an organizational model for addressing errors and problems based on support, treating staff members justly and fairly, and shared accountability and responsibility among the organization and its staff. The organization takes responsibility for errors caused by the design and operation of its system whereas staff are accountable for their contribution to errors and problems and take responsibility for accurately reporting errors and system vulnerabilities.

Table 3 provides some characteristics of each environment type and how they relate to critical event response.

DISCUSSION

This article began by saying that many factors come together in often unpredictable ways to affect critical event response. The challenge is for teams to be aware of and manage them as effectively as possible. Returning to the beginning scenario, how factors discussed in 4 major areas (see **Fig. 3**) came together in this event is considered

The patient was a 55-year-old, 75-kg woman with a prior inferior MI and breast cancer, to undergo reconstructive breast (left) surgery after a complete mastectomy. The procedure was delayed for more than 4 hours because of OR scheduling problems *(this can cause a number of other problems like fatigue and impatient and rushed staff)* and staff availability *(although not stated, it is possible that someone not scheduled had to fill in; this person may not have had a chance to become familiar with the case, may be fatigued, or—if an itinerant clinician—possibly is unaware of processes used at this site, location of emergency equipment, and so forth)*. The surgical resident was extremely anxious to begin *(likely placing pressure on others to rush and increasing team stress level)* and the anesthesiology attending had not had an expected break for lunch 2 hours earlier *(hunger and fatigue can impair cognitive functioning and overall performance)*. Anesthesia was induced without problem and the patient was prepped and draped. Just prior to incision, the patient's heart rate suddenly began to drop *(a sudden and unexpected critical event can catch clinicians by surprise and impair initial reactions[30])*.

The first year clinical anesthesia resident (CA1) *(a relatively inexperienced clinician)* increased the patient's oxygen to 100% and administered 0.2-mg atropine *(0.3-mg less than recommended in advanced cardiac life support [ACLS] guidelines[31])*. A nurse summoned the anesthesiology attending STAT *(recognition by a team member of the need for additional resources/expertise)*. A minute later the attending arrived and administered 10-μg epinephrine as the heart rate continued to drop. The surgical resident complained about the delay *(distracting and adding pressure and not contributing to the response as a member of the team; there is some question as to whether the resident is aware that a critical event is occurring [ie, lack of situation awareness])* as the anesthesia attending instructed the CA1 to perform chest compressions while he administered an arrest dose of epinephrine *(escalation of therapy in response to a refractory condition)*, asked the OR nurse to call for help (recognition that help is needed and the task—getting help—is appropriately delegated to a team member),

Table 3
Primary environment characteristics affecting critical event response

Environment Type	Primary Characteristics	Possible Effects on Response
Physical	Lighting	Low lighting may make it difficult to see patient and/or equipment, drug labels, and supplies
	Temperature	Hot or cold temperatures may • Make it difficult for clinicians to focus on patients, symptoms, and treatment and slow their cognitive processing • Affect a patient's metabolism and clotting factors, thereby affecting the efficacy of drugs administered • Be desired or required for certain types of events (eg, treat burn patients or deal with premature newborns)
	Weather and terrain	Wind and/or precipitation or inhospitable terrain may make it difficult to • Manipulate materials and supplies (eg, syringes) • Set up tents or access equipment • Establish/maintain a sterile field
	Clutter or insufficient work space	A cluttered or crowed work space may make it difficult • For enough clinicians to have access to the patient or move freely without risk of injury • To locate and/or move needed equipment • To observe some symptoms or cues (eg, blood on the floor due to massive hemorrhage; kinked hoses) • Maintain a sterile field
	Noise	Unnecessary or loud noise may • Make it difficult for clinicians to concentrate, retain information in working memory, and recall prospective memory tasks at the right time[26] • Impair clinicians' ability to communicate or coordinate with each other • Add to a sense of chaos and increase everyone's stress levels

(continued on next page)

Table 3 (*continued*)		
Environment Type	**Primary Characteristics**	**Possible Effects on Response**
Work	Misplaced, unavailable, or difficult to obtain equipment	Slows, impairs, or prohibits correct clinician response
	Nonstandardized equipment	Equipment of the same type that is configured or operates differently used within the facility (eg, different makes and models of anesthesia machines in different ORs) increases the likelihood of clinician error,[27] especially during critical event response.
	Processes, procedures, and workflow	• Those that are well-thought out, logical, streamlined, and are consistent with operational demands tend to facilitate response[28]—those that are not tend to impair response.[28]
	Insufficient personnel	Insufficient numbers of personnel or personnel with needed specialties can impair correct or timely critical event response.
	Team training and cognitive aids for critical events	Availability of such training and aids can improve clinician coordination and response to critical events.[29]
Cultural	Rigid hierarchies	Can impair communication and coordination across team members with different specialty backgrounds
	Learning institution	Data regarding critical events and event response are collected and analyzed, so interventions to reduce the likelihood of events occurring and improve response
	Just culture vs blame culture	• Just culture values identification of errors/problems in critical event response and their root causes so they can be addressed • In a blame culture, clinicians are more likely to hide or not report errors or problems with event response—thus, they go unaddressed and may be repeated

(*continued on next page*)

Environment Type	Primary Characteristics	Possible Effects on Response
Table 3 *(continued)*		
Community and national	Rigid hierarchical structures	Can impair communication and coordination across individuals with different training, genders, ages, etc.
	Heavy emphasis on community or national pride	Can inhibit sharing, publicizing, or even acknowledging critical event occurrences and/or errors or problems with critical event response, thereby depriving the institution and others from learning from each other in addressing the problems
Certification and regulatory	Punitive actions for errors/poor response to critical events	• May be appropriate in cases where institutions have not identified problems, conducted root cause analyses, and implemented effective interventions • May cause institutions to hide or minimize occurrence of critical events or problems with response
	Work with institutions to support development of learning and just culture environment	Increases likelihood that critical events and problems with response will be acknowledged, systemic and individual root causes will be identified, and effective interventions will be implemented in a supportive and fair manner

Content in this table is not comprehensive.
Data from Refs.[26–29]

and started to set up an epinephrine infusion *(implementing ACLS recommended actions)*. The very short CA1 complied, but even standing on her tiptoes had trouble administering compressions at an adequate depth *(she does not think to ask for and no one thinks to get the CA1 a stool to stand on—it is common to not think of simple things like this when under time pressure and stress)*. The surgical attending kept entering and exiting the OR asking about progress *(distracting, not contributing to the response as a member of the team; apparent lack of situation awareness that a critical event is occurring)*, as the anesthesiologist first inadvertently programmed the epinephrine infusion at 1500-μg/min (the maximum dosing for dopamine) and then immediately corrected to 10-μg/min *(common type of cognitive error when under stress)*. A circulating nurse, on his own volition, went and obtained a crash cart *(good anticipation of need but lack of team leadership, communication, and coordination)*; the anesthesiologist was unaware that it was available *(treatment options, such as external pacing, not remembered and team communication breakdown)* as he worked frantically to address the patient's increasing bradycardia and switch with the CA1 in providing compressions *(anesthesiologist clearly is under stress although remembered that the compressor—the CA1—needed to be relieved but did not elicit help of other present team members to be compressors, however)*.

The surgical resident continued to ask how much longer it would be until the patient was stabilized *(again, distracting and adding pressure, not contributing a member of the team and lack of situation awareness)*. While doing chest compressions, the anesthesiologist noticed that the anesthetic gas was still on *(very delayed identification of situation that should have been addressed earlier—note that no critical event checklist is being used)* and he immediately told the CA1 to turn it off. He then told the surgical resident that they needed to focus on stabilizing the patient and postpone the reconstructive surgery *(anesthesiologist demonstrating some leadership in suggesting appropriate action)*.

This scenario is similar to many that occur daily. The anesthesiology attending is the leader in managing the event, as is often the case with OR critical events, but demonstrates leadership erratically. He does ask the circulating nurse to get help, tells the CA1 to administer compressions, and tells the surgical resident that the patient should be stabilized and procedure postponed. He is not using personnel resources (eg, surgical resident and attending, nurses) effectively, however. It is possible that this lack of leadership is due to stress related limits of cognitive bandwidth (ie, overtaxed working memory, system 2 thinking, and problem solving) and/or it could be related to team member personality factors that operate in the background to negatively affect the ability of individuals present to cohere as a team. It also could reflect something about the cultural environment of the institution, such as rigid role expectations across professions (anesthesiology, surgery, and nursing).

The anesthesiologist appears to lack awareness of the overall situation and is largely reactive—response and work flow appear chaotic with several errors and actions being missed. Cognitive overload such as this is common in critical events[3] and is exacerbated by things such as fatigue, hunger, and having to monitor a junior trainee (CA1). A critical event checklist could have helped the anesthesiologist better structure response and avoid the errors but only if (1) a checklist had been available and (2) the anesthesiologist remembered to use it—use of such cognitive aids during critical events can require the involvement of others as readers, so, again, the anesthesiologist would have had to lead by assigning tasks and roles to team members.

Recommendation: when in the leader role during a critical event, clinicians should clearly announce that a critical event is occurring as soon as it is apparent and assign roles to available team members, get additional help early (when it is needed), and, when appropriate, consider primarily trying to direct the actions of others so as to better be able to monitor the entire situation. Research examining aviation accidents found that events were handled more successfully when the captain was in charge of managing the event and running the checklist than when actively trying to fly the plane and manage the event concurrently.[32]

SUMMARY

Clinicians should not discount the insidious ways that a multitude of factors can come together and create a perfect storm that impedes effective critical event response. Changes to even 1 or 2 factors (fatigue or not, extra people available to help or not, and checklist available or not) can change the response process and outcome completely. The bradycardia event of today is not necessarily going to evolve and resolve as the bradycardia event that was masterfully managed last week. Always be thinking about ways that you can prepare for the things you can control, minimize potential vulnerabilities as much as possible, and appreciate and accommodate for your own natural limitations—cognitive, physical, emotional, and otherwise.

ACKNOWLEDGMENTS

The authors wish to thank Dr Genie Heitmiller, Dr Alex Hannenberg, and Dr Anna Clebone who provided feedback on the clinical examples in this article. The authors are especially grateful for the help and suggested edits to the scenario provided by Drs Heitmiller and Hannenberg. Nonetheless, any errors or deficiencies that remain are our own.

REFERENCES

1. Burian BK, Barshi I, Dismukes K. The challenge of aviation emergency and abnormal situations. NASA/TM—2005—213462. Moffett Field (CA): NASA Ames Research Center; 2005.
2. Kahneman D. Attention and effort. Engelwood Cliffs (NJ): Prentic-Hall, Inc; 1973.
3. Dismukes RK, Kochan JA, Goldsmith TE. Flight crew errors in challenging and stressful situations. Aviat Psychol Appl Hum Factors 2018;8(1):35–46.
4. Dismukes RK. Introduction. In: Dismukes RK, editor. Human error in aviation. Farnham Surrey (England): Ashgate; 2010. p. xiii–xxiv.
5. Woods DD, Dekker S, Cook R, et al. Behind human error. Farnham Surrey (England): Ashgate; 2010.
6. Kahneman D. Thinking, fast and slow. New York: Farrar, Straus and Giroux; 2011.
7. Schneider W, Shiffrin RM. Controlled and automatic human information processing: I. detection, search, and attention. Psychol Rev 1977;84(1):1–66.
8. Marewski JN, Gigerenzer G. Heuristic decision making in medicine. Dialogues Clin Neurosci 2012;14(1):77–89.
9. Berner ES, Graber ML. Overconfidence as a cause of diagnostic error in medicine. Am J Med Qual 2008;121(5, Supplement):S2–23.
10. Didwania A, Chadha V, Didwania A, et al. Improving medical decision making in real time: teaching heuristics and bias. Society of General Interenal Medicine Web Site. Available at: https://www.sgim.org/File%20Library/SGIM/Resource%20Library/Meeting%20Handouts/SGIM/2010/WC02——Teaching-Heuristics-in-Real-Time.pdf.
11. Groopman JE. How doctors think. Boston: Houghton Mifflin; 2007.
12. Dismukes RK. Prospective memory in workplace and everyday situations. Curr Dir Psychol Sci 2012;21(4):215–20.
13. Dodhia RM, Dismukes RK. Interruptions create prospective memory tasks. Appl Cogn Psychol 2009;23(1):73–89.
14. Loukopoulos LD, Dismukes RK, Barshi I. The multitasking Myth: handling complexity in real-world operations. Farnham Surrey (England): Ashgate; 2009.
15. Gaba DM, Maxwell M, DeAnda A. Anesthetic mishaps: breaking the chain of accident evolution. Anesthesiology 1987;66(5):670–6.
16. Sokol DK. Waking up to the effects of fatigue in doctors. BMJ 2013;347:f4906.
17. Parker JB. The effects of fatigue on physician performance - an underestimated cause of physician impairment and increased patient risk. Can J Anaesth 1987;34(5):489–95.
18. Ghazali DA, Breque C, Sosner P, et al. Stress response in the daily lives of simulation repeaters. A randomized controlled trial assessing stress evolution over one year of repetitive immersive simulations. PLoS One 2019;14(7):e0220111.

19. Easdown LJ, Banerjee A, Weinger MB. Simulation to assess human responses to critical events. In: Lee JD, Kirlik A, editors. The Oxford handbook of cognitive engineering. New York: Oxford University Press; 2013. p. 336–51.
20. Gillespie BM, Gwinner K, Fairweather N, et al. Building shared situational awareness in surgery through distributed dialog. J Multidiscip Healthc 2013;6:109–18.
21. Hu YY, Arriaga AF, Peyre SE, et al. Deconstructing intraoperative communication failures. J Surg Res 2012;177(1):37–42.
22. Buljac-Samardzic M, Doekhie KD, van Wijngaarden JDH. Interventions to improve team effectiveness within health care: a systematic review of the past decade. Hum Resour Health 2020;18(1):2.
23. O'Dea A, O'Connor P, Keogh I. A meta-analysis of the effectiveness of crew resource management training in acute care domains. Postgrad Med J 2014; 90(1070):699–708.
24. Fanning RM, Goldhaber-Fiebert SN, Udani AD, et al. Crisis resource management. In: Levine AI, DeMaria S Jr, Schwartz AD, et al, editors. The comprehensive textbook of healthcare simulation. New York: Springer; 2013. p. 95–107.
25. Raghunathan K. Checklists, safety, my culture and me. BMJ Qual Saf 2012;21(7): 617–20.
26. Cannon-Bowers JA, Salas E, editors. Making decisions under stress. Washington, DC: American Psychological Association; 1998.
27. Cooper JB, Newbower RS, Long CD, et al. Preventable anesthesia mishaps: a study of human factors. Anesthesiology 1978;49(6):399–406.
28. Burian BK. Factors affecting the use of emergency and abnormal checklists: implications for current and NextGen operations. Moffett Field (CA): NASA Ames Research Center; 2014. NASA/TM-2014-218382.
29. Hart EM, Owen H. Errors and omissions in anesthesia: a pilot study using a pilot's checklist. Anesth Analg 2005;101(1):246–50.
30. Kochan JA, Breiter EG, Jentsch F. Surprise and unexpectedness in flying: database reviews and analyses. Proc Hum Factors Ergon Soc Annu Meet 2004;48(3): 335–9.
31. Liu LA. ACLS bradycardia Algorithm. ACLS training center Web site. 2019. Available at: https://www.acls.net/acls-bradycardia-algorithm.htm. Accessed April 23, 2020.
32. Jentsch F, Barnett J, Bowers CA, et al. Who is flying this plane anyway? What mishaps tell us about crew member role assignment and air crew situation awareness. J Cogn Eng Decis Mak 1999;41(1):1–14.

High-Fidelity Simulation Education and Crisis Resource Management

Amanda R. Burden, MD

KEYWORDS

- Anesthesiology/education • Crisis management • Medical education • Feedback
- Mannequins • Performance improvement • High-fidelity simulation • Patient safety

KEY POINTS

- High-fidelity simulation is used to teach the skills and techniques that are essential to managing critical events in anesthesiology.
- This article explores high-fidelity simulation in anesthesiology education and provides strategies for its use to improve management of critical events.
- High-fidelity simulation is useful in teaching both technical (diagnostic and procedural) and nontechnical (communication and professionalism) skills, including crisis resource management skills.

ANESTHESIOLOGY LEADERSHIP IN CRISIS MANAGEMENT AND HIGH-FIDELITY SIMULATION

Simulation-based education in health care emerged as the result of efforts by anesthesiologists to improve crisis management and patient safety. Over the past few decades, medical schools and hospitals have launched simulation programs and credentialing, and governing bodies now require the addition of simulation to both educational and certification processes.[1–3]

Critical event management requires significant discipline and knowledge. Anesthesiologists must have a full understanding of physiology and pathophysiology and the ability to function and make decisions in dynamic settings.[1,2] An important hallmark of anesthesiology is that the anesthesiologist must be responsible for clinical decision making and for ensuring execution of the plan. Successful crisis management requires that anesthesiologists diagnose and treat problems in an extremely short time frame. It is also essential for anesthesiologists to maintain vigilance so they can identify and respond to emergency situations. Mastering these skills, along with the ability to communicate with and lead a team, must be developed and continually improved

Clinical Skills and Simulation, Cooper Medical School of Rowan University, Cooper University Healthcare, CMSRU Simulation Center, 201 South Broadway, Camden, NJ 08103, USA
E-mail address: burdena@rowan.edu

Anesthesiology Clin 38 (2020) 745–759
https://doi.org/10.1016/j.anclin.2020.08.006
1932-2275/20/© 2020 Elsevier Inc. All rights reserved.

throughout a career. There are many forms of simulation education, all of which are excellent educational modalities. This article focuses on high-fidelity simulation education, which allows learners an opportunity to learn and practice key elements of managing crises in anesthesiology.[1–3] Additional approaches to simulation education are discussed elsewhere in this edition (Article 3).

MANAGING ANESTHESIA CRISES

Crisis resource management (CRM) is a model created to address aviation safety by helping crews identify and resolve serious events in flight and specifically focuses on interpersonal communication, leadership, and decision making.[1,3] David Gaba and his team adapted CRM from aviation to address anesthesiology crises in the 1990s and incorporated simulation education to teach and refine physician performance during crises.[3] An important CRM goal is to focus the attention of individuals and the entire team to recognize and respond to crises early and to improve the responses of the individuals and the team to the evolving events. Although medical knowledge and technical skills are essential components of patient care in a crisis, nontechnical skills, such as leadership, communication, and situational awareness, are equally critical for the safe care of patients.[1–3] To manage the crisis effectively, anesthesiologists must manage the full situation.[1,2]

CRISIS RESOURCE MANAGEMENT PRINCIPLES

Gaba and colleagues[2] describe a set of principles and actions that comprise effective CRM (**Table 1**). These principles comprise actions that focus the team on effective coordination of all activities in response to an evolving event. It is expected that many of these principles (eg, effective communication) will carry over to routine activities in ways that will prevent the initiation of an event. Key CRM principles are briefly discussed here.[1–5]

KNOW THE ENVIRONMENT

It is essential to know what available resources are available. These resources may include knowing who is available at what time to provide assistance, what equipment is available, and where important equipment is stored.[2,3]

Table 1 Crisis resource management key points	
Dynamic Decision Making	**Team Management**
Know the environment	Call for help early
Anticipate and plan	Designate leadership
Use all available information	Establish role clarity
Allocate attention wisely	Distribute the workload
Mobilize resources	Communicate effectively
Use cognitive aids	Establish situational awareness and a shared mental model

Adapted from Gaba DM, Fish KJ, Howard SK, et al. Crisis management in anesthesiology. Elsevier Health Sciences; 2014. p. 25-53; with permission.

ANTICIPATE AND PLAN

Vigilance is an essential tenet of the practice of anesthesiology; anticipating and planning are critical elements of that practice. The team should plan for and consider the risks of a particular patient or procedure for the occurrence of a crisis during the anticipated procedure in advance.[2]

SITUATION AWARENESS

While caring for patients, especially during crises, it is vital to maintain awareness of every change that occurs to the patient and the environment.[2–5] It is also important to be aware of the actions of others involved in the care of the patient. This is termed situation awareness.[2–5]

CALL FOR HELP EARLY

Calling for help is the sign of a strong and competent anesthesia professional. It is critical to call for help at the earliest sign of a problem in order to make a difference in the patient's care, especially in an emergency, or if the patient's condition is deteriorating and the patient is unresponsive to interventions. Another person can see things that might have been missed and can provide additional physical resources. Another person can also help discuss the patient's diagnosis and treatment options.[2,3,6–8] Calling for help early is particularly challenging for many professionals because it could be construed as a sign of indecision or weakness, when it is instead a sign of expertise and can be the critical element that determines success or failure in preventing an adverse outcome.[2,3]

DESIGNATE LEADERSHIP

A well-functioning team must have an effective leader who takes command of the team, coordinates the overall event management, communicates about the patient's status, and distributes the required work.[2,7] To fulfill these leadership functions, the anesthesiologist must be knowledgeable, must have excellent technical and nontechnical skills, and must remain calm and organized. An important part of the leader's role is to articulate the full plan so the team has a shared mental model of the patient's situation and plan and will be able to follow the plan. The team leader must also be open to input and suggestions from other members of the team because they may have critical information. Being open to receiving communication from the other team members helps ensure that all available information about the patient can be incorporated into the plan. Disagreement about the optimal care elements should not be about who is right, but about what is right for the patient.[1–3,7,8]

FOLLOWERSHIP

Other members of the team must be mindful followers. They must pay clear attention to the leader's information and requests and must also be actively engaged so they can provide any missing information. Although it is the leader's job to coordinate the patient's care, everyone on the team is responsible for the patient's safety.[1–3,6–8]

USE ALL AVAILABLE INFORMATION

There is usually a great deal of information that must be understood and integrated during a critical event, which adds to the complexity of anesthetic care.[2,3,6,7]

Information must be collected from all possible sources and that information must be considered and discussed with the team. It is crucial to deliberately investigate diagnoses that may not fit the leader's original view of the situation to avoid missing the correct diagnosis and fixating on one that was incorrect and formed too early.[1-4,6-8]

ESTABLISH ROLE CLARITY

Efforts to create a well-functioning team must begin before an emergency arises and the team is needed. These efforts require the cooperation of all of the team members. All team members must be clear about their individual roles and responsibilities. Team members who know the plan and their roles are more likely to be effective, and team coordination is then easier. Crises are usually tense situations; repeated, periodic briefings by the leader can help calm team members and focus them on caring for the patient.[1-4,6,7]

ALLOCATE ATTENTION WISELY

The leader and the team must continue to reassess the critically ill patient at all times. It is also important to alternate between focusing on details and focusing on the big picture. At times, specific details require full focus (eg, a difficult intubation), but the leader must then refocus attention on the larger patient situation as that situation evolves. While the leader is focused on accomplishing a specific task, at least 1 anesthesia professional, if available, should be assigned to monitor the patient's condition. If the evolving crisis becomes more demanding, the required tasks may become more complex and additional resources may be needed.[1-3,6-8]

DISTRIBUTE THE WORKLOAD

There are many tasks that must be completed in a crisis, often at the same time. The leader should prioritize and delegate these whenever possible.[2,7] The leader should define the tasks, verify that they are properly performed, and review changes in the patient's situation. If possible, the team leader should remain free of manual tasks in order to observe, gather information, and delegate tasks.

MOBILIZE RESOURCES

Mobilizing resources requires time and planning. Ideally, the team leader should request needed resources as early as possible, so they arrive in time to help. The knowledge and skills of the team leader and team members are the most important resources. Whatever resources are available should be used; a crisis should not be managed alone when there are people available who could help or equipment that could be used.[2,7]

COMMUNICATE EFFECTIVELY

Managing crises requires clear, closed-loop communication. Team members should be addressed directly and should confirm that the information was heard. This approach allows all team members to know what is happening and what is planned as the crisis evolves.[2,3,7]

USE COGNITIVE AIDS

There are many forms of cognitive aids or checklists. These checklists are especially important for situations when things must be done in a specific order and skipping a step could lead to disastrous results (eg, omitting dantrolene while treating a patient with malignant hyperthermia).[2,3] Cognitive aids are discussed in more detail in Article 5.

ESTABLISH SITUATIONAL AWARENESS AND A SHARED MENTAL MODEL

Anesthesia is a dynamic process; this is especially true during crises. The team's understanding of the patient's condition may be precisely right at one moment and wrong at the next. Such changes may dramatically alter the approach to management. The leader and the team must continually investigate and discuss any changes and how those affect the presumed diagnosis and treatment plan.[2–4]

HIGH-FIDELITY SIMULATION AND CRISIS MANAGEMENT

High-fidelity simulation, which is able to realistically replace real-patient experiences in a safe environment, is an excellent technique to teach and learn the elements of CRM and how to incorporate them into practice.[2] Various types of simulators are used to train and assess different levels of learners, including mannequin simulators, human cadaver or animal models, computer-based simulation, haptic and/or virtual simulation, as well as simulation using standardized patients. Many of these methods are discussed in Article 3. Simulation has emerged as a valued educational methodology and is now an accepted part of training, assessment, and research in all levels of medical education from novice to experienced board-certified physician.[1–4,9,10]

ADULT LEARNING THEORY AND HIGH-FIDELITY SIMULATION

Creating a successful simulation program requires that faculty understand and implement key themes of adult learning theory.[10,11] Adult learners are self-directed and goal oriented; they expect to learn information that is timely, relevant, and practical. Adults learn through experiential learning, which is characterized by a cycle of experiences, reflection, conceptualization, and experimentation (feeling, reflecting, thinking, doing).[12] Deliberate practice, which allows learners to repeatedly address errors through immediate and constructive feedback, is an important tool for adult learners.[11] Simulation creates an environment of experiential learning where learners can engage in deliberate practice to learn and ultimately master technical and nontechnical skills.[1–4,6,13].

High-fidelity simulation provides an ideal environment for anesthesiologists to learn from mistakes, build on prior knowledge, and reflect on performance to learn to safely manage crises.[1–3,9,10,13–15] The simulation environment with faculty-guided feedback and debriefing sessions allows learners to reflect on their experiences and discuss crisis management concepts in a setting without the stress of patient care. Best-practice features in simulation have been described by McGaghie and colleagues[10,15] (**Table 2**). These features allow learners to use simulation as a tool so they may repeatedly practice procedures and other fundamental aspects of patient care[12] (**Fig. 1**).

Anesthesiologists use high-fidelity simulation to acquire a wide variety of skills, including procedural skills, clinical reasoning and judgment, teamwork, crisis management, and professionalism.[1–3,13] By allowing learners to engage in high-risk procedures in a safe environment where they can later reflect on their performance and consider how to improve, simulation provides an excellent opportunity to teach adult

Table 2 Best-practice features of effective simulation education	
Feature	**Benefits**
Feedback	Allows learner to reflect to review performance and identify errors and opportunities to improve
Deliberate practice	Allows learner to repeatedly practice skills to gain expertise and improve
Curriculum	Simulation sessions should be integrated into an overarching curriculum
Outcome measurement	Defined, measurable outcomes are important for learners at all levels
Simulator validity and fidelity	Choose the best type of simulator or simulation tool to fit learning objectives
Skill acquisition and maintenance	Sessions should allow learners to repeatedly perform different skills so they can build on and develop expertise and increase retention
Mastery learning	Simulation sessions should be designed so learners are able to address errors and practice skills to gain expertise
Transfer to practice	Sessions should allow learners to transfer skills to patient care
Team training	Simulation provides an ideal opportunity to allow teams to train together
High-stakes testing	Simulation environments may be standardized and used for high-stakes testing
Instructor training	Faculty development and education in reflective learning techniques and debriefing skills is essential in creating a robust simulation program
Educational and professional context	Sessions must be relevant to practice and provide realistic representations of the patient care environments

Adapted from Refs.[10,15]

learners. This point is particularly true for rare cases and crises that learners may not have had the opportunity to experience during residency but must be able to identify and manage as practicing anesthesiologists. Some of these events are discussed in detail later in this article, such as lost airway, intraoperative cardiac arrest, obstetric hemorrhage, and oxygen supply failure.[1–3,13,14]

PRINCIPLES OF SIMULATION EDUCATION

The opportunity for learners to engage in deliberate practice (DP) is an essential feature of simulation-based education.[11] DP is an educational paradigm designed to improve skill development. It involves repeated and consistent practice where learners review their performance through feedback. DP is a key element of expertise development in many different domains, including sports, commerce, performing arts, science, and writing. DP use has led to more effective skill acquisition and accomplishment than experience or intellectual ability. DP is an effective method to allow learners to acquire and hone both technical and nontechnical skills.[10,11,15] High-fidelity simulation–based education creates an environment in which learners can

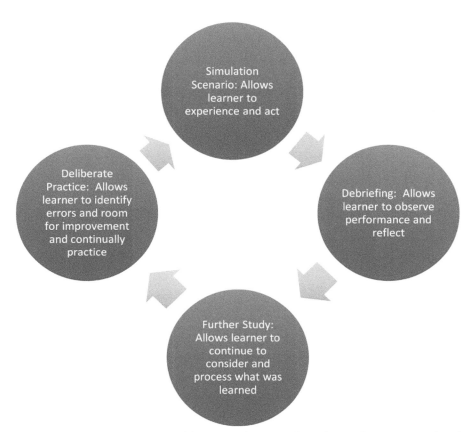

Fig. 1. Simulation and experiential learning. Elements of simulation that correspond with the adult learning cycle. (*Adapted from* Counselman FL, Carius ML, Kowalenko T, et al. The American Board of Emergency Medicine Maintenance of Certification Summit. J Emerg Med 2015; 49:722–8; with permission).

use DP to practice. Through this core feature of simulation education, they are able to make mistakes and errors and learn from those experiences in a setting that is safe for both them and their patients. They are able to work with mentors and instructors to receive feedback about those mistakes so they can learn from them and achieve proficiency.[1,10,11,15] DP has served as an effective educational method to teach several procedures and to teach nontechnical skills. Examples of skills that have been successfully taught using simulation with DP include central line placement, lumbar puncture, intubation, communication during a code, and handovers or transfers of care.[15–22]

SIMULATION AND PERFORMANCE IMPROVEMENT

Simulation allows repeated practice in an environment that encourages reflection through debriefing sessions and thus provides a powerful performance improvement modality.[10,15] McGaghie and colleagues[15] explored the use of simulation to improve and enhance performance of technical procedures. Others have shown that simulation is successful as a tool to teach and analyze teamwork, especially in complex situations.[7,8] Simulation allows for the design of specific clinical experiences, standardization of content, and the opportunity for interactive learning in a clinical setting without patient risk.[23]

Nontechnical Skills

Nontechnical skills are critically important for managing crises and for managing teams. High-fidelity simulation provides an excellent platform to teach these skills. Simulated environments allow health care teams to enact clinical decisions and explore the decision-making process within an environment where communication and team dynamics can be carefully reviewed and considered.[1–3,14]

Team Performance

High-fidelity simulation education provides an ideal platform for teamwork and CRM education. Mannequin simulators provide complex physiologic platforms that, when combined with the ability to create realistic clinical environments, allow the health care team to learn to work through different clinical scenarios together. They are able to then debrief the experience with an expert facilitator to identify what went well and where the team needs to improve.[1–3,14,24]

CHARACTERISTICS OF SCENARIOS FOR USE IN CRISIS RESOURCE MANAGEMENT TRAINING

To be useful for CRM training, simulation scenarios usually have special requirements:

- Interaction with the team is required. Members of the rest of the clinical team should be fully interactive, whether played by real clinicians in combined-team training or by actors or standardized patients acting in the roles.
- Interpersonal challenges are presented. Scenarios should be created that require handling interpersonal issues, whether between clinical team members, with patients, or with the patient's family.
- Requires operationalizing backup plans. It is important to present scenarios where trainees need to move beyond their expected plan to a plan B or even plan C, D, or even E, and so on. For the scenario, the initial responses should not be sufficient to solve the problem.
- Learners must look beyond an initial diagnosis. It is important for learners to explore differential diagnoses beyond their initial impressions. Simulation allows for the presentation of confounding information that suggests several possible causes for the patient's problem.
- Scenarios cover a variety of different problems. Some scenarios may be primarily about technical and environment challenges, such as power failure, oxygen failure, or faulty equipment. Some may be about ethical challenges. Others can relate to specific infrequently faced clinical conditions requiring special responses (eg, cardiac arrest scenarios).

FOUNDATIONS OF BEHAVIORAL CHANGE

Performance improvement efforts require collaboration from all stakeholders (patients, providers and leaders) to be successful. Anesthesiologists' desire to improve the quality of care has been essential to achieving the goal of sustained positive outcomes. Moreover, effective data collection, identification of areas of opportunity for improvement, and the necessary support to create and sustain local and/or systemic change have been key elements of the specialty's dramatic progress in advancing quality and safety.[25] Those tasked with managing performance improvement efforts must recognize that changing external circumstances such as environments, processes, or resources does not automatically render changes in behavior.[25]

ANESTHESIOLOGY LEADERSHIP IN PERFORMANCE IMPROVEMENT

Anesthesiology has long led efforts in medicine to methodically and scientifically review and evaluate patient safety to identify opportunities and solutions to improve patient care. Dr Ellison (Jeep) Pierce[26] kept careful accounts of "anesthesia accidents," and anesthesiologists were early adopters of critical incident analysis applied to health care crises.[6,26] Through the creation of the American Society of Anesthesiologist (ASA) Committee on Patient Safety and Risk Management, the Anesthesia Patient Safety Foundation, and the Anesthesia Quality Institute, anesthesiology has emerged as a leader in efforts to improve quality and patient safety.[27,28] Through these efforts, several anesthesia-specific registries were created to capture data nationally for the purpose of identifying and disseminating best practices.[28] The ASA has been a leader in identifying and exploring opportunities and strategies to improve performance through quality improvement programs. In addition, the American Board of Anesthesiology (ABA) requires demonstration of practice improvement as part of ongoing Maintenance of Certification in Anesthesiology (MOCA) and, in 2010, proposed simulation as a mechanism to satisfy this requirement.[29,30]

THE AMERICAN SOCIETY OF ANESTHESIOLOGISTS

The ASA created the Workgroup on Simulation Education in 2004. The workgroup established a framework that programs could follow to provide high-fidelity simulation–based educational courses that would be appropriate for attending physician anesthesiologists. In 2006, this workgroup surveyed ASA members to identify their educational needs. Of the 1350 physicians who responded, most (81%) were interested in continuing medical education (CME) programs that were simulation based. A large percentage (77%) of physicians who responded to the survey indicated they preferred CME education involving simulation and that it offered more powerful benefits than those offered by conventional sessions and lectures. Physician ASA members also responded that the most important features of simulation-based education were a realistic mannequin (77%), a high instructor/student ratio (76%), and that the simulated environment be realistic (69%). Videotaping of their performance (51%) and the opportunity for multidisciplinary training (50%) were identified less frequently by ASA members as necessary components of simulation-based CME. In addition, 71% indicated that they wanted their performance to be assessed. These respondents expressed their desire to use these sessions to improve their practice.[29,30] At the same time, the ASA created the ASA Committee on Simulation Education to encourage and promote the availability of superior simulation-based education for its members. The committee developed program criteria that were required to receive endorsement from the ASA. These criteria include requirements for faculty development, robust educational sessions, and space requirements. Programs meeting these criteria were endorsed beginning in 2009 and the ASA Simulation Education Network (SEN) was established.[31,32] Soon after the SEN was established, the ABA charged the committee with developing a simulation-based educational program that would provide the opportunity for physician anesthesiologists to reflect on and improve their performance. In 2010, simulation became an approved component of the part 4 MOCA requirement.[29,30]

THE AMERICAN BOARD OF ANESTHESIOLOGY

The part 4 (improving medical practice) component of MOCA requires that physicians engage in an educational activity that allows them to reflect on their practice and identify opportunities where they can improve. In 2010, the ABA officially incorporated simulation courses designed by the ASA Simulation Committee as part of this part 4 MOCA component.[29,30] These high-fidelity mannequin simulation courses were selected for several reasons: (1) high-fidelity simulation–based education has established that it is able to engage participants and encourage them to reflect on their performance and change practice and behavior,[2,3,7–10,15,21,22] a feature that allows participants to assess their own performance and identify gaps in their practice; (2) through high-fidelity simulation, participants have the opportunity in a simulated environment to practice managing rarely occurring clinical scenarios that are high risk for patients; and (3) participants are able to view video recordings of their performance after the simulation sessions so they can reflect on opportunities for improvement.[1,9,15] These MOCA simulation courses allow learners to explore and learn about the medical and technical skills that are essential in the management of perioperative challenges and crises. Participants are able to practice and review skills required for managing health care teams, assessing the situation, and arriving at a decision to appropriately manage an evolving crisis. The courses are videotaped with debriefing sessions following each scenario. This ability to engage in video review and debriefing allows for reflection on performance in the scenarios and identification of specific areas in their practice that could be improved. Participants then submit their plans for practice to the ASA and spend the following 90 days working to execute these changes. Following this effort, the learners report about the results of this effort. The physician anesthesiologists are encouraged to discuss their successes as well as barriers they faced. This simulation program is not an examination; instead, it is an opportunity to engage in a personal practice assessment and improvement activity and be recognized with CME and MOCA credit.[29–32]

The physicians who have participated in the MOCA simulation courses have reported that it has been a positive educational experience. Findings from postcourse surveys reveal that 95% of participants reported that they would recommend simulation to their colleagues, and 98% indicated that the course was relevant to their practice. Students who completed the courses indicated that the most important aspect was that the courses were relevant to their practice. Surveys conducted a few months following the courses identified that 95% of participants had successfully completed the proposed changes in their practice that they recognized during the courses.[29]

The practice plans created by several physicians who participated in these courses were impressive in their scope and were responsible for considerable impact on their departments and hospital systems. The practice improvement plans and subsequent follow-up reports for more than 1800 participants were reviewed; often challenging barriers were overcome. The students in these courses reported that they had accomplished far more than they initially anticipated. Often specific benefits for patients related to improving teamwork and communication skills were accomplished. Other examples included disseminating management guidelines, such as emergency manuals, across departments and even hospital networks. Interprofessional collaboration was remarkable in many instances. In addition, one of the course participants reported that he used intraosseous insertion techniques he learned during a MOCA simulation course to save a patient's life.[31–33]

A team of anesthesiologists from 12 academic institutions received funding from the Agency for Healthcare Research and Quality (AHRQ) to study whether mannequin-based simulation courses can be standardized and whether those courses can consistently show how skilled physicians would manage medical emergencies.[34] Expert raters were able to review videos of the scenarios and rate both the technical and nontechnical performance of the subjects. Study results indicated that roughly 80% of essential management steps were accomplished and three-quarters of the subjects performed at a middle level or better. Study results also revealed approaches to improve safety in the perioperative setting. Importantly, a key finding was that it was very meaningful when the subject requested assistance from another physician. Researchers noted that another physician entering the scenario to assist the subject almost always led to improvement in the care in the scenario. The study was not designed to identify the proficiency or ability of the subject physicians. Still, the scenarios did allow the investigators to study the range of performance during the simulated representations of recognized crises. The research team further identified that recognition of the need to escalate treatment when the initial therapy was not sufficient, using evidence-based approaches to treatment, and communicating directly with other members of the patient-care team presented other important practice improvement opportunities.[31,34]

MEDICAL MALPRACTICE

Medical malpractice insurance companies are important stakeholders in the advancement of simulation-based education. These companies have incorporated simulation into many different programs, all of which use simulation to motivate performance improvement education and behaviors among physicians and the health care team. In 2001, the Risk Management Foundation of the Harvard Medical Institutions (CRICO), which serves as the malpractice insurer for Harvard-affiliated health care institutions, introduced courses that used simulation education to provide education in CRM and provided insurance premium discounts for anesthesiologist participants in these courses.[35,36] Analyses of malpractice activity conducted after the program had run for many years revealed that there were fewer claims and there was a reduction in overall claims costs. Building on this early success, CRICO offered a larger discount to physician anesthesiologists enrolled in the program. This reduction in claims was significant enough that CRICO asked simulation experts to establish similar courses for physicians in other disciplines. They also established a team training course for operating room teams.[35,36] Other malpractice insurance companies have identified the benefits of simulation training and have incorporated it into premium reduction programs for their insured physicians.[35–38]

SIMULATION AND FUTURE RESEARCH

The AHRQ, the Anesthesia Patient Safety Foundation, Foundation for Education and Research in Anesthesia (FAER), and many other specialty societies and foundations have provided funding to encourage further research in simulation education. Educational and research societies have also held consensus conferences where experts in simulation education and research were invited to collaborate, discuss, and generate additional important topics to investigate.[39] The increasing focus on simulation-based education has led to the creation and improvement of these simulation centers. Many medical specialty societies other than the ASA and ABA are focused on studying best practice in simulation education and creating guidelines. Several societies have created guidelines for accreditation of simulation programs and centers. The American College of Surgeons (ACS) created a consortium of ACS-accredited Education Institutes. These programs offer global opportunities for collaboration, research, and access to resources, with the goal of improving surgical care and practice using simulation education. Information detailing their application process and a list of the other accredited centers is available on the ACS Web site.[40] The mission of the inter-professional and multidisciplinary Society for Simulation in Healthcare (SSH) is to facilitate excellence in health care education, practice, and research through simulation. SSH is another society that accredits simulation programs and is focused on expanding and improving simulation education and research.[41]

SUMMARY

Physician performance improvement along with skill maintenance has become increasingly important to the public. Conventional conferences and other didactic activities that provide CME often do not lead to the changes and improvement in practice that the public expects.[42–44] These more traditional instructional approaches have seldom provided a forum where practice improvement and transfer from learning to clinical environments was demonstrated.[45]

There is a long history of anesthesiologists' efforts to review practice and identify errors and opportunities to change behavior and improve practice. Their role in identifying and advancing CRM in health care is an important part of this effort. Through their specialty certification board and academic societies, they have also created educational sessions and a culture that encourages and deliberately engages in performance improvement. Physician anesthesiologists were pioneers in the patient safety movement and established programs designed to identify and address errors that led to patient harm even when there was resistance to this idea and long before it became accepted and important to the medical community and among the population. Anesthesiologists have contributed significant innovations to the practice of medicine that have improved patient care and enhanced patient safety. Simulation is one of these considerable contributions.

ACKNOWLEDGMENTS

The Anesthesia Patient Safety Foundation Safety Scientist Career Development Award (PI A. R. Burden), Rochester, MN and (R18HS026158, PI M.B. Weinger) from the Agency for Healthcare Research and Quality, Washington, DC.

REFERENCES

1. Gaba DM. The future vision of simulation in health care. Qual Saf Health Care 2004;13(Suppl 1):i2–10.

2. Gaba DM, Fish KJ, Howard SK, et al. Crisis management in anesthesiology. Philadelphia: Elsevier Health Sciences; 2014.

3. Burden A. The history of crises and crisis management in anesthesia: prevention, detection, and recovery. Int Anesthesiol Clin 2020;58(1):2–6.

4. Gaba DM, Howard SK, Small SD. Situation awareness in anesthesiology. Hum Factors 1995;37(1):20–31.

5. Endsley MR. Design and evaluation for situation awareness enhancement. In: Proceedings of the human factors society, 32nd annual meeting, Santa Monica, CA, October 24–28, 1988. p. 97–101.

6. Cooper JB, Newbower RS, Long CD, et al. Preventable anesthesia mishaps: a study of human factors. Anesthesiology 1978;49:399–406.

7. Salas E, Wilson KA, Murphy CE, et al. Communicating, coordinating, and coop-
erating when lives depend on it: tips for teamwork. Jt Comm J Qual Patient Saf
2008;34:333–341.
8. Salas E, DiazGranados D, Klein C, et al. Does team training improve team performance? a meta-analysis. Hum Factors 2008;50:903–33.
9. Cooper JB, Taqueti VR. A brief history of the development of mannequin simulators for clinical education and training. Postgrad Med J 2008;84(997):563–70.
10. McGaghie WC, Issenberg SB, Petrusa ER, et al. A critical review of simulation
based medical education research: 2003-2009. Med Educ 2010;44(1):50–63.
11. Ericsson KA. Deliberate practice and the acquisition and maintenance of expert
performance in medicine and related domains. Acad Med 2004;79(10 Suppl):
S70–81.
12. Kolb D. Experiential Learning: experience as the source of learning and development. Upper Saddle River (NJ): Prentice-Hall; 1984.
13. Sinz E. Simulation-based education for cardiac, thoracic, and vascular anesthesiology. Semin Cardiothorac Vasc Anesth 2005;9(4):291–307.
14. Gaba DM, Howard SK, Fish K, et al. Simulation-based training in anesthesia crisis
resource management (ACRM): a decade of experience. Simul Gaming 2001;
32(2):175–93.
15. McGaghie WC, Issenberg SB, Cohen ME, et al. Does simulation-based medical
education with deliberate practice yield better results than traditional clinical education? a meta-analytic comparative review of the evidence. Acad Med 2011;
86(6):706.
16. Barsuk JH, McGaghie WC, Cohen ER, et al. Simulation-based mastery learning
reduces complications during central venous catheter insertion in a medical
intensive care unit. Crit Care Med 2009;37:2697–701.
17. Cohen ER, Feinglass J, Barsuk JH, et al. Cost savings from reduced catheter-
related bloodstream infection after simulation-based education for residents in
a medical intensive care unit. Simul Healthc 2010;5:98–102.
18. Burden AR, Torjman MC, Dy GE, et al. Prevention of central venous catheter-
related bloodstream infections: is it time to add simulation training to the prevention bundle? J Clin Anesth 2012;24(7):555–60.
19. Issenberg SB, McGaghie WC, Gordon DL, et al. Effectiveness of a cardiology review course for internal medicine residents using simulation technology and
deliberate practice. Teach Learn Med 2002;14:223–8.
20. Wayne DB, Didwania A, Feinglass J, et al. Simulation-based education improves
quality of care during cardiac arrest team responses at an academic teaching
hospital. Chest 2008;133:56–61.
21. Burden AR, Pukenas EW, Deal ER, et al. Using simulation education with deliberate practice to teach leadership and resource management skills to senior resident code leaders. J Grad Med Educ 2014;6(3):463–9.
22. Pukenas EW, Dodson G, Deal ER, et al. Simulation-based education with deliberate practice may improve intraoperative handoff skills: a pilot study. J Clin
Anesth 2014;26(7):530–8.
23. Gordon JA, Wilkerson WM, Shaffer DW, et al. "Practicing" medicine without risk:
Stu- dents' and educators' responses to high- fidelity patient simulation. Acad
Med 2001;76:469–72.
24. Howard SK, Gaba DM, Fish KJ, et al. Anesthesia crisis resource management
training: teaching anesthesiologists to handle critical incidents. Aviat Space Environ Med 1992;63(9):763–70.

25. Solomons NM, Spross JA. Evidence-based practice barriers and facilitators from a continuous quality improvement perspective: an integrative review. J Nurs Manag 2011;19(1):109–20.
26. Pierce EC Jr. The 34th rovenstine lecture. 40 years behind the mask: safety revisited. Anesthesiology 1996;84:965–75.
27. Stoelting RS. Patient safety: a brief history. In: Ruskin K, Stiegler M, Rosenbaum S, editors. Quality and safety in anesthesia and perioperative care. New York (NY): Oxford University Press; 2016. p. 3–15.
28. Dutton RP, Dukatz A. Quality improvement using automated data sources: the anesthesia quality institute. Anesthesiol Clin 2011;29:439–54.
29. McIvor W, Burden A, Weinger MB, et al. Simulation for maintenance of certification in anesthesiology: the first two years. J Contin Educ Health Prof 2012;32:236–42.
30. Steadman RH, Berry AJ, Coursin DB, et al. Simulation and MOCA®: ASA and ABA perspective, after the first three years. ASA Newsletter 2013;77(8):30–2.
31. Weinger MB, Burden AR, Steadman RH, et al. This is not a test! misconceptions surrounding the maintenance of certification in anesthesiology simulation course. Anesthesiology 2014;121(3):655–9.
32. Steadman RH, Burden AR, Huang YM, et al. Practice improvements based on participation in simulation for the maintenance of certification in anesthesiology program. Anesthesiology 2015;122(5):1154–69.
33. Anson JA. MOCA saves a life [letter]. ASA Newsletter 2013;77(1):47.
34. Weinger MB, Banerjee A, Burden AR, et al. Simulation-based assessment of the management of critical events by board-certified anesthesiologists. Anesthesiology 2017;127(3):475–89.
35. Hanscom R. Medical simulation from an insurer's perspective. Acad Emerg Med 2008;15:984–7.
36. CRICO/RMF. Clinician resources: team training. Available at: https://www.rmf.harvard.edu/Clinician-Resources/Article/2014/OR-Team-Training-Incentive. Accessed April 15, 2020.
37. The doctors company resources. Available at: http://www.thedoctors.com. Accessed April 17, 2020.
38. DeMaria S, Levine A, Petrou P, et al. Performance gaps and improvement plans from a 5-hospital simulation programme for anaesthesiology providers: a retrospective study. BMJ Simul Technol Enhanc Learn 2017. https://doi.org/10.1136/bmjstel-2016-000163. bmjstel-2016.
39. Dieckmann P, Phero JC, Issenberg SB, et al. The first research consensus summit of the society for simulation in healthcare: conduction and a synthesis of the results. Simul Healthc 2011;6(Suppl):S1–9.
40. American College of Surgeons, Division of Education Accredited Education Institutes, Enhancing patient safety through simulation. Available at: http://www.facs.org/education/accreditationprogram/requirements.html. Accessed April 21, 2020.
41. Society for simulation in healthcare council for accreditation of healthcare simulation programs informational guide for the accreditation process from the SSH council for accreditation of healthcare simulation programs. Available at: https://www.ssih.org/Credentialing/Accreditation. Accessed April 21, 2020.
42. Davis D, O'Brien MA, Freemantle N, et al. Impact of formal continuing medical education: do conferences, workshops, rounds, and other traditional continuing education activities change physician behavior or health care outcomes? JAMA 1999;282(9):867–74.

43. Counselman FL, Carius ML, Kowalenko T, et al. The American board of emergency medicine maintenance of certification summit. J Emerg Med 2015;49: 722–8.
44. Holmboe ES, Wang Y, Meehan TP, et al. Association between maintenance of certification examination scores and quality of care for medicare beneficiaries. Arch Intern Med 2008;168:1396–403.
45. Steadman RH. Improving on reality: can simulation facilitate practice change? Anesthesiology 2010;112(4):775–6.

Alternatives to High-Fidelity Simulation

Megan Delisle, MD, MPH, MSc[a], Alexander A. Hannenberg, MD[b],*

KEYWORDS

- Low-fidelity simulation • Telesimulation • Role playing • Facilitation • Debriefing

KEY POINTS

- Simulation-based education is the preferred method for training health care professionals on how to manage critical events.
- Significant barriers related to training, technology, and time prevent widespread uptake of high-fidelity simulation.
- Alternatives to high-fidelity simulation include in situ simulation, classroom-based simulation, telesimulation, observed simulation, screen-based simulation, and game-based simulation.
- Alternatives to onsite expert debriefing include teledebriefing, scripted debriefing, and within-group debriefing.
- Alternatives to high-fidelity simulation and onsite expert facilitation should be tailored to match local resources for the purpose of increasing access to this model of training.

INTRODUCTION

The global need for high-quality health care and patient safety has never been higher. Critical events in health care represent an important source of preventable patient morbidity and mortality. Managing critical events requires a unique skill set for which health care professionals need to receive formal training and have opportunities to practice. This skill set demands proficiency in technical skills (eg, resuscitation drugs) and nontechnical skills (eg, closed loop communication). Because both are essential for success, learning taskwork and teamwork in critical event training is intrinsically synergistic.

For more than two decades, health care has made enormous investments in the promotion of high-fidelity, high-technology, simulation training often citing the examples of high-reliability organizations, such as aviation and nuclear power, despite that these industries differ in fundamental ways from the health care industry.

[a] Department of Surgery, University of Manitoba, 347-825 Sherbrook Street, Winnipeg, Manitoba R3T 2N2, Canada; [b] Ariadne Labs, Tufts University School of Medicine, 401 Park Drive, 3 West, Boston, MA 02115, USA
* Corresponding author.
E-mail address: ahannenberg@ariadnelabs.org

Anesthesiology Clin 38 (2020) 761–773
https://doi.org/10.1016/j.anclin.2020.08.001
1932-2275/20/© 2020 Elsevier Inc. All rights reserved.
anesthesiology.theclinics.com

BARRIERS TO SIMULATION-BASED EDUCATION

High-fidelity simulation training is underused in health care because of three main types of barriers (the three Ts): (1) cost of technology, (2) availability of time, and (3) access to trained simulation facilitators. Existing simulation centers deliver an intensive and powerful training experience but number fewer than 500 in the United States with a health professional workforce of 10 million. These figures describe a profound and intrinsic barrier to scaling delivery of high-fidelity simulation. Training adults preferentially uses experiential, rather than didactic, teaching approaches of which simulation is an exemplar.[1] Simulation-based training involves three key activities (**Table 1**).

The value and success of this training is highly dependent on the role of the simulation educator who facilitates the design and delivery of the training and the debriefer who manages the reflection phase of the training. These roles may or may not be combined, but both are essential. Although the barriers presented by the technology and time demands of high-fidelity simulation may be most obvious, the scarcity of trained simulation educators may be the most impactful obstacle, limiting the delivery of a wide range of simulation training.

ALTERNATIVES TO HIGH-FIDELITY SIMULATION

There exist several alternatives to simulation center–based education that can help overcome barriers related to the three Ts. At the core of creating an effective simulation experience is maintaining fidelity, defined as "the degree to which the simulation replicates the real event and/or workplace; this includes physical, psychological, and environmental elements" (**Table 2**).[2] It is psychological fidelity that is believed to be the most essential for effective learning because it creates emotional engagement that is associated with improved retention and long-term recall.[3–6] Thus, cheaper, easier, and faster alternatives to simulation center–based education that maintain psychological fidelity have the potential to be equally effective and can help lower the barriers. These alternatives to high-fidelity simulation are often referred to as low-fidelity simulation, but this nomenclature is misleading because these alternatives still maintain a high degree of psychological fidelity. The terms "low-technology" or "low-barrier" simulation are preferred because they more accurately reflect the three Ts framework. This has important implications for health care organizations with limited resources who recognize the value of this type of training and are looking for alternatives to increase accessibility.

The training, technology, and time required to deliver simulation center–based education at scale is often prohibitive. Several lower technology alternatives have been designed to overcome these barriers (**Table 3**).[5] Limited application of these approaches has been undertaken for some time in health care, most notably in mock

Table 1 Key activities in simulation-based training	
Briefing (ie, Prebriefing)	Introduces activities, learning objectives, and promotes psychological safety
Simulation scenario	Emulates real-life experience, creates emotional engagement in the learning exercise, and illustrates the learning objectives
Debriefing	A framework for learners to reflect on the experience of the scenario and learn

Table 2 Types of fidelity in simulation-based education	
Physical fidelity	The degree to which the simulation duplicates the appearance and feel of the real system
Environmental fidelity	The extent to which the simulator duplicates motion cues, visual cues, and other sensory information from the environment
Psychological fidelity	The degree to which the trainee perceives the simulation to be a believable surrogate for the trained task

Data from Beaubien JM, Baker DP. The use of simulation for training teamwork skills in health care: how low can you go? Qual Saf Health Care. 2004 Oct; 13(Suppl 1): i51–i56.

codes, malignant hyperthermia simulations, and, more recently, in obstetric hemorrhage. The potential application and scale of this training is far from reaching its potential, especially with respect to nontechnical skill learning objectives.

In Situ Simulation

Rationale
In situ simulation is an alternative to simulation center–based education that is used in settings with limited access to dedicated simulation centers. In situ simulation often allows for the delivery of education at the point of care, which can substantially decrease the travel time commitment required for facilitators and participants. An additional benefit of in situ simulation is that it often reveals unrecognized system weaknesses and for these reasons it is often used as part of quality improvement initiatives.[12,13]

Experience with in situ simulation training for critical events
Few examples of randomized controlled trials exist evaluating the benefits of in situ simulation. Sørensen and colleagues[14] conducted one of the landmark trials comparing in situ simulation with off-site simulation center–based training for the clinical management of emergency caesarean section and a postpartum hemorrhage in Copenhagen, Denmark. They randomized multiprofessional teams of midwives, nurses, anesthetists, and obstetricians and gynecologists and evaluated differences in knowledge, patient safety attitudes, stress levels, team performance, and organizational impact. Overall, there were no differences in outcomes between the two groups except that the in situ simulation group did have more ideas and suggestions for changes at the organizational level and rated the simulation as more authentic.[15] Several additional examples of nonrandomized studies have been published demonstrating the benefits of in situ simulation in training interprofessional operating room teams in the management of critical events.[16]

Considerations
In situ simulation often introduces highly realistic simulated equipment, devices, and drugs in the training environment to increase the level of fidelity and emotional engagement of participants. There have been reports of inadvertent migration of these props into real patient care leading to some concerns over the safety of in situ simulation.[17] Numerous recommendations designed to mitigate this risk have been identified.[18] Trained facilitators are still required to design and conduct training, and guide participants' reflection on their simulation experience.[19] However, the amount of time required to travel to off-site simulation centers is eliminated, making the commitment more manageable for participants and facilitators. Although this is a benefit in some

Table 3 Alternatives to high-fidelity simulation	
In situ simulation	Simulation that "takes place in the actual patient care setting/environment in an effort to achieve a high level of fidelity and realism."[2]
Classroom-based simulation (eg, role playing, mental practice, part-task trainers)	Simulation that is conducted without technological requirements in virtually any environment, including classrooms, meeting spaces, and conference halls. Examples include role playing, mental practice, and part-task trainers: Role playing, commonly also referred to as table-top simulation, uses "written scripts and oral presentations to present and review clinical scenarios without hands-on learning."[2] Mental practice is the process of mentally rehearsing an action to enhance performance.[7] Part-task trainers are "models that represent a part or region of the human body such as an arm, or an abdomen. Such devices may use mechanical or electronic interfaces to teach and give feedback on manual skills such as IV insertion, ultrasound scanning, suturing, etc. They are generally used to support procedural skills training; however they can be used in conjunction with other learning technologies to create integrated clinical situations."[2]
Telesimulation	"A process by which telecommunication and simulation resources are utilised to provide education, training and/or assessment to learners at an off-site location, where an off-site location is considered a distant site that would preclude education, training and/or assessment without the use of telecommunication resources."[8]
Observed simulation	Observing live or prerecorded video interactions of real people in a simulated or real clinical environment without the use of telecommunication.[9,10]
Screen-based simulation	The use of mobile tablets, smartphones, computer screens, and other screen-based devices to allow the end-user to interact with a simulated clinical environment using a keyboard, mouse, joystick, or other input device.[2]
Game-based simulation	The application of game design elements, such as rules, scoring mechanisms, and leaderboards, to simulation-based education with the goal of teaching participants skills or knowledge in an interactive way that is also enjoyable.[2] Can range from high-technology platforms, such as virtual games, to low-technology applications, such as role playing and tabletop games.[11]

Data from Refs.[2,7–11]

respects, the tradeoff is an increased likelihood of cancellation, reportedly as high as 43% because of staff being diverted to clinical care demands.[20]

Classroom-Based Simulation

Rationale
Role playing, mental practice, and part-task trainers are alternatives to high-fidelity and in situ simulation that do not need any sophisticated equipment thereby reducing the technological barriers to simulation-based education. They can be delivered in

virtually any environment, including classrooms, meeting spaces, and conference halls. When conducted in close proximity to clinical environments, they can be integrated into regular meeting times to reduce disruptions to clinical duties and improve participation for facilitators and participants.[21] Although role playing is ideal for team-based simulations, mental practice is a variant that allows individual team members to engage in cognitive rehearsal and has been shown to improve performance in health care.[22] For additional technical skills training, part-task trainers are introduced to deliver simulation in settings where access to technology is restricted while still giving participants the opportunity to practice the skills they are being taught. Part-task trainers include basic manikins, household items, and patient monitor emulators and are often available at a fraction of the cost of high-technology, computer-driven manikins. They are used in conjunction with other props to recreate a low-technology simulated immersive clinical environment within any setting.[2] There is empirical evidence suggesting that despite lower environmental and equipment fidelity, these types of simulations can result in effective learning with no significant disadvantage relative to high-technology, simulation center–based education.

Experience with classroom-based simulation training for critical events

There is some experience that has demonstrated the benefits of role playing, mental practice, and part-task trainers in managing critical events. Role playing is a recommended strategy for training operating room personnel on how to appropriately use the World Health Organization Safe Surgery Checklist.[23] For example, role playing was a part of the state-wide implementation strategy of the Safe Surgery Checklist in South Carolina that resulted in a 22% decline in postoperative mortality.[24,25]

Louridas and colleagues[22] conducted a randomized controlled trial where 20 senior surgical trainees were randomized to either conventional training or mental practice for advanced laparoscopic skills. Technical skills were assessed during a crisis scenario where the patient developed an anaphylactic reaction midprocedure. Residents randomized to the mental practice group were able to better maintain their performance under stressful conditions.

An example of successful use of part-task trainers that is familiar to many health care professionals is the simple torso manikin used in most Advanced Cardiac Life Support (ACLS) classroom-based training programs. These types of low-technology models have also been successfully used to bring simulation-based education to low-resource settings. For example, the Helping Babies Breath program uses a simple infant manikin to enhance delivery room resuscitation. Implementation of the program resulted in significant reductions in neonatal deaths in Tanzania, India, and Kenya.[26]

Considerations

Role playing, mental practice, and part-task trainers are forms of experiential learning that are used for a variety of individual- and team-based simulations. Although minimal equipment is needed and delivery is accommodated in a variety of easily available locations, trained facilitators often are still required to assist with the development of scenarios and guiding participants through the briefing and debriefing portions of the simulations. With respect to preparation for such exercises, there are resources available to support local development of training scenarios.[27,28]

Telesimulation and Observed Simulation

Rationale

Active participation in simulation scenarios is generally limited to four to five participants, who are usually alternating between active participation in the scenario and observation of fellow participants. To deliver simulation-based education at scale, an increase in the capacity of simulation scenarios is desperately needed. For these reasons, alternatives to active participatory simulation, such as telesimulation and observed simulation, have emerged. These types of simulations still meet the needs of adult learners because they are based on real-life scenarios that elicit emotional responses and psychological engagement.[29–32] A recent systematic review and meta-analysis compared the learning achievement in observed versus active participatory simulation and found similar learning outcomes between the two modalities when participants were provided with specific learning objectives and debriefing guidance.[9]

Experience with telesimulation and observed simulation training for critical events
Telesimulation has only recently emerged as an alternative to high-fidelity simulation center–based training.[8] McCoy and colleagues[33] published the first randomized controlled trial using this modality. Thirty-two fourth-year medical students were randomized to standard high-fidelity simulation or telesimulation training in casualty triage. The telesimulation group watched the standard high-fidelity group participate in an immersive, simulation center–based scenario via a live television Internet connection. After the scenario, both groups participated in a debriefing. The authors reported no significant differences in satisfaction or gains in knowledge between the two groups.[33]

Observed simulation has been used to successfully train anesthesia trainees how to manage critical events in the operating room. For example, Bong and colleagues[34] randomized 37 anesthesia trainees to either active participation or observation of high-fidelity simulation training where they were required to manage three different pediatric anesthesia emergencies. The authors found both groups achieved equivalent levels of nontechnical performance. Lai and colleagues[35] conducted a similar randomized controlled trial among anesthesia trainees and concluded active participation was not superior to observation for training crisis resource management. Vortman[36] recently published her innovative educational intervention where high-fidelity simulation-based scenarios of massive hemorrhage in the operating room were recorded and played to a large audience during monthly staff meetings followed by a debrief. This was part of a larger quality improvement initiative where more than 150 operating room personnel were trained to enhance performance with massive transfusion protocols. Without this innovative strategy to deliver high-volume simulation training, more than 45 simulation sessions would have been required.

Considerations
Telesimulation and observed simulation require trained debriefers to guide participants through the briefing and debriefing portion of the simulation but debriefers are not necessarily required to design the scenario. Telesimulation makes use of high-speed Internet and advanced telecommunication resources to connect observers to offsite simulations. This reliance on technology can result in limitations in some low-resource settings and creates susceptibility to occasional malfunction.[37–39] Observation of recorded simulation videos can greatly reduce the telecommunication resources required because only basic audiovisual equipment and a suitable area for viewing and debriefing are needed.

Screen-Based Simulation

Rationale
There are several advantages to screen-based simulations. First, they can have built-in feedback mechanisms and automated facilitation capabilities that reduce the need for availability of trained facilitators. The virtual platforms can often host a large number of end-users simultaneously and allow for either individual or team-based

simulations. Participants can usually access these resources remotely on demand and can engage in synchronous or asynchronous use. This allows flexibility in scheduling that allows participants to complete the required training on their own timetable without competing with clinical duties.

Experience with screen-based simulation training for critical events

Screen-based simulation has been embraced for ACLS training in which it is typically used as an individual activity with an emphasis on technical skills, that is, ACLS treatment algorithms.[40] In a randomized controlled trial of 65 third-year medical students, those randomized to screen-based ACLS simulation training had a significantly shorter time to defibrillate ventricular tachycardia compared with those without training (112 vs 150 seconds, respectively; $P<.05$).[41] Anesthesia SimSTAT is another, similar, example focused on clinical aspects of managing operating room critical events. In this example, a series of virtual clinical scenarios are available on a computer screen and the participant is an avatar on the screen that can practice managing critical events. Although the learning effectiveness of this specific platform has never been validated, similar screen-based simulations for the management of noncritical events in anesthesiology have proven to be effective.[42] The application of this training technology to nontechnical skills, such as teamwork and communication, critical factors in optimizing performance, is more limited.

Considerations

Screen-based simulation is a versatile application that can accommodate a large number of users while minimizing the time required to participate and the need for experienced facilitators. Although some commercially available platforms exist (eg, Anesthesia SimSTAT), many institutions may find a need for their own platforms for specific, local training needs.[43] In this situation, the considerable production costs and technical expertise required can limit access to this otherwise effective method.

Game-Based Simulation

Rationale

Game-based simulations aim to make participants feel increasingly motivated and engaged in the learning process with the hope of overcoming barriers related to participants' competing time demands.[44] Game-based simulations are versatile and suitable for individual-level simulations (eg, single player virtual games) and team-based simulations (eg, multiplayer virtual games, role playing, tabletop games) and technical and nontechnical skills training. An advantage unique to virtual platforms is that some have built-in automated facilitation capabilities thus alleviating the need for available and trained facilitators.

Experience with game-based simulation training for critical events

Several examples of game-based simulations exist for training critical events, but few that have been empirically evaluated.[45] Kurenov and colleagues[46] developed *Burn Center*, an interactive, video game–based simulation designed to improve the technical and nontechnical skills required for trauma surgeons, nurses, therapists, and other emergency services to effectively triage and resuscitate burn victims of mass casualty disasters. Only brief preliminary results are available demonstrating "a positive correlation between training with *Burn Center* and performance in a traditional lectured course."[46] Rouse and colleagues[47] created *Emergency Birth!*, a video game–based simulation that aims to reinforce safe emergency obstetric birth practices among rural traditional birth attendants. They piloted it among 50 traditional rural birth attendants in Mexico and found participants reported it to be a feasible and effective method for teaching.[47] Taekman and colleagues collaborated with the United States Army and Virtual Heros, a state-of-the-art virtual games developer, to create *3DiTeams*, a multiplayer online game-based simulation that aims to improve teamwork and communication in the management of critical events in health care.[48] The learning effectiveness of this platform has never been evaluated. Although it is mostly virtual game-based simulations that have been described in the published literature, there is anecdotal evidence to support the use of low technology and tabletop game-based simulations in the training of critical event management. More formal evaluation and dissemination of these platforms are warranted given their increased accessibility and sustainability in most settings.

Considerations

Game-based simulations are an excellent way of improving participant motivation and engagement, but there are several important details that should be considered before local implementation. Several examples of game-based simulations exist for training critical events, but the evidence to support their learning effectiveness is limited. Although there are some available games that have been produced and are used "out of the box," many educators interested in using game-based simulation find themselves having specific needs that require them to develop platforms de novo. This often requires expert guidance and resources. Although some virtual platforms have built-in facilitation capabilities, some do not. The use of no-technology team games unrelated to the clinical world, such as Legos, will require advanced skills to translate the game's learning points to real-life practice scenarios. Finally, depending on the platform used to deliver the game-based simulation, access to audiovisual equipment, high-speed Internet, and expert onsite facilitators may be required.

ALTERNATIVES TO EXPERT ONSITE FACILITATION

An important limitation to adopting most of the previously listed alternatives to high-fidelity simulation is the reliance on expert facilitators to design and implement simulations exercises. Even when the simulation scenario is acquired from expert sources, the need to conduct briefs and debriefs remains essential. To overcome the scarcity of trained debriefers, several alternatives to expert onsite debriefing have been developed (**Table 4**).

Teledebriefing

Rationale

Using teledebriefing, debriefers at remote locations can observe participants in their simulation and then lead them through a reflection on their actions. This is a good

Table 4 Alternatives to expert onsite debriefing	
Teledebriefing	Use of telecommunication and audiovisual equipment to connect participants to debriefers at an off-site location
Scripted debriefing	Allows new debriefers to step into the role using scripts with debriefing prompts that are curated in advance by expert facilitators for the simulated scenario
Within-group debriefing	Provides debriefing scripts directly to small groups of participants with clear instructions on how the debriefing should be conducted without a debriefer present

Data from Refs.[49,50]

option for settings with limited access to trained facilitators but with access to resources for simulation scenarios and high-speed Internet connection. It is also advantageous from the perspective of debriefers because it can minimize the burdens of travel, cost, and time away from other responsibilities.

Experience with teledebriefing in training for critical events

Ahmed and colleagues[51] randomized emergency medicine residents to either teledebriefing or on-site debriefing after 11 high-fidelity, crisis resource management simulations. The simulation scenarios were conducted in a simulation center equipped with audiovisual equipment that allowed the remote debriefer to watch the participants interactions in real time. Teledebriefings were conducted using an iPhone camera that was plugged into a large television monitor to maximize participants visualization and allow the debriefer to see participants during the debriefing. All debriefings were conducted by expert debriefers who had completed 1-year fellowships in medical simulations. Participants rated their perception of debriefing effectiveness using the validated Debriefing Assessment for Simulation in Healthcare.[52] The authors found that both the on-site debriefing and teledebriefing were rated as "consistently effective/very good." A similar study by Ikeyama and colleagues[53] with 16 fellows from the departments of anesthesia and intensive care found 87% of participants rated teledebriefing at least as effective as on-site debriefing.

Considerations

Similar to telesimulation, teledebriefing relies on high-speed Internet to connect participants and debriefers at separate locations. This requires the areas for simulation scenarios be equipped with the appropriate resources to allow debriefers to have a good view of the interactions that are occurring. For these reasons, this modality is susceptible to technological failures, particularly when connecting to remote areas with reduced capabilities. Although teledebriefing can increase access to trained debriefers and decrease the travel, time and costs incurred by debriefers, this can put additional strain on trained facilitators whose skills are often already in high demand in their local settings.[54] Teledebriefing is logistically challenging when used across time zones. When used across cultures, differences in communication style, hierarchy, and decision-making may limit facilitators ability to connect with participants during the debriefing, which is critical to creating a safe space for learning and open and honest reflection. Despite these potential limitations, there is a small but growing body of evidence supporting the use of this modality to improve access to trained debriefers.[39,51]

Scripted and Within-Group Debriefing

Rationale

Scripted and within-group debriefing are alternatives that are used in settings with limited access to trained debriefers. They have many advantages. Scripted debriefing allows educators new to simulation-based education to step into role with graded exposure. Having debriefing prompts designed by experts ahead of time based on the learning objectives can assist in transitioning into a more independent debriefer over time. Although this approach is limited by the extent to which the expert can fully anticipate the events in the simulation, it does allow for a graduated approach that is helpful in areas where mentorship and peer coaching are limited. In some settings, there may not be anyone to take on the task of debriefer or the participant number may be too large relative to the number of debriefers available. Use of prerecorded clinical scenarios and subsequent small-group breakout sessions for within-group debriefing allows a much larger capacity for participants that can increase the scalability of simulation-based education.

Experience with scripted and within-group debriefing in training for critical events
Although there are a limited number of studies evaluating scripted and within-group debriefing, the slowly accumulating body of evidence is promising. For example, Cheng and colleagues[55] conducted a multicenter randomized controlled trial to assess the effectiveness of using debriefing scripts for new debriefers without formal training in teaching Pediatric Advanced Life Support. All participants were required to manage a 12-month-old infant with hypotensive shock. Participants were randomized to undergo a debriefing with a new debriefer that functioned with or without a script. The authors found that teams with scripted debriefers demonstrated more gains in knowledge, clinical performance, and team leadership. Boet and colleagues[56] randomized 40 operating room teams to either within-group or instructor-led debriefing. All teams were required to manage a simulated operating room crisis. The authors found that within-group and instructor-led debriefing resulted in improvements in team performance without any significant difference between groups.

Considerations
Many simulation societies recommend facilitators have advanced training in simulation design and debriefing before stepping into this role.[57] One of the most important reasons for this recommendation is to mitigate the risk of psychological distress in participants caused by either activities in simulated scenarios or triggering recall of personal traumatic events. Seasoned facilitators often have the skills and experience to identify these situations early, steer the conversations back to safety, and identify participants that may need additional attention after the debriefing. This is an important concern that might represent a shortcoming of scripted and within-group debriefing and needs additional investigation despite the promising results of early studies on the learning outcomes. Scripted debriefing requires new debriefers to step into this role with little experience. Although Cheng and colleagues's work demonstrates positive results, it does not capture the challenge of recruiting new debriefers to this daunting role.[58] Within-group debriefing can overcome the need to recruit new debriefers, but a better understanding of the psychological risks and strategies to mitigate this in the absence of trained facilitators are needed.

FUTURE DIRECTIONS FOR ALTERNATIVES TO HIGH-FIDELITY SIMULATION IN CRITICAL EVENT TRAINING

Many critical events in health care are a source of preventable morbidity and mortality that is overcome with appropriate training. Simulation-based education is ideal for training health care professionals how to manage critical events but is too often inaccessible, especially at a frequency required to prevent knowledge decay. Several alternatives to simulation center–based, immersive simulation and expert facilitation were introduced in the previous sections that are used to reduce the training, technology, and time required to deliver simulation-based education. Each of these variations have evolved to overcome specific limitations and the ideal permutation depends on the local setting. Although the available evidence on the learning effectiveness of many of these novel approaches is encouraging, it is variable. Nonetheless, it is likely their use will continue to spread as the demand for cheaper, faster, and easier yet still effective simulation-based education for training in critical event management and other skills increases.

DISCLOSURE

This work is supported by American Hospital Association Team Training.

REFERENCES

1. Knowles MS, Holton EF, Swanson RA. The adult learner: the definitive classic in adult education and human resource development. 8th edition. New York: Routledge Taylor & Francis Group; 2015.
2. Lopreiato JO. Healthcare simulation dictionary. Rockville (MD): Agency for Healthcare Research and Quality; 2016. Publication No. 16(17)-0043.
3. Tyng CM, Amin HU, Saad MNM, et al. The influences of emotion on learning and memory. Front Psychol 2017;8:1454.
4. Norman J. Systematic review of the literature on simulation in nursing education. ABNF J 2012;23(2):24–8.
5. Nippita S, Haviland MJ, Voit SF, et al. Randomized trial of high- and low-fidelity simulation to teach intrauterine contraception placement. Am J Obstet Gynecol 2018;218(2):258.e1–11.
6. Finan E, Bismilla Z, Whyte HE, et al. High-fidelity simulator technology may not be superior to traditional low-fidelity equipment for neonatal resuscitation training. J Perinatol 2012;32(4):287–92.
7. van Meer JP, Theunissen NCM. Prospective educational applications of mental simulation: a meta-review. Educ Psychol Rev 2009;21(2):93–112.
8. McCoy CE, Sayegh J, Alrabah R, et al. Telesimulation: an innovative tool for health professions education. AEM Educ Train 2017;1(2):132–6.
9. Delisle M, Ward MAR, Pradarelli JC, et al. Comparing the learning effectiveness of healthcare simulation in the observer versus active role: systematic review and meta-analysis. Simul Healthc 2019;14(5):318–32.
10. Delisle M, Pradarelli JC, Panda N, et al. Methods for scaling simulation-based teamwork training. BMJ Qual Saf 2020;29(2):98–102.
11. McCoy L, Lewis JH, Dalton D. Gamification and multimedia for medical education: a landscape review. J Am Osteopath Assoc 2016;116(1):22–34.
12. Yajamanyam PK, Sohi D. In situ simulation as a quality improvement initiative. Arch Dis Child Educ Pract Ed 2015;100(3):162–3.
13. Barbeito A, Bonifacio A, Holtschneider M, et al. In situ simulated cardiac arrest exercises to detect system vulnerabilities. Simul Healthc 2015;10(3):154–62.
14. Sørensen JL, van der Vleuten C, Rosthøj S, et al. Simulation-based multiprofessional obstetric anaesthesia training conducted in situ versus off-site leads to similar individual and team outcomes: a randomised educational trial. BMJ Open 2015;5(10):e008344.
15. Sørensen JL, Navne LE, Martin HM, et al. Clarifying the learning experiences of healthcare professionals with in situ and off-site simulation-based medical education: a qualitative study. BMJ Open 2015;5(10):e008345.
16. Owei L, Neylan CJ, Rao R, et al. In situ operating room-based simulation: a review. J Surg Educ 2017;74(4):579–88.
17. Raemer D, Hannenberg A, Mullen A. Simulation safety first: an imperative. J Surg Simul 2018;5:43–6.
18. Tool Kit/Resources – Foundation for Healthcare Simulation Safety. Available at: https://healthcaresimulationsafety.org/tool-kit-resources/. Accessed April 11, 2020.
19. Guise J-M, Mladenovic J. In situ simulation: identification of systems issues. Semin Perinatol 2013;37(3):161–5.

20. Kurup V, Matei V, Ray J. Role of in-situ simulation for training in healthcare: opportunities and challenges. Curr Opin Anaesthesiol 2017;30(6):755–60.
21. Joyner B, Young L. Teaching medical students using role play: twelve tips for successful role plays. Med Teach 2006;28(3):225–9.
22. Louridas M, Bonrath EM, Sinclair DA, et al. Randomized clinical trial to evaluate mental practice in enhancing advanced laparoscopic surgical performance. Br J Surg 2015;102(1):37–44.
23. Ariadne Labs. Safe Surgery Checklist Implementation Guide. 2015. Available at: https://www.ariadnelabs.org/wp-content/uploads/sites/2/2018/08/safe_surgery_implementation_guide__092515.012216_.pdf. Accessed February 15, 2020.
24. Berry WR, Edmondson L, Gibbons LR, et al. Scaling safety: the South Carolina Surgical Safety Checklist experience. Health Aff (Millwood) 2018;37(11):1779–86.
25. Haynes AB, Edmondson L, Lipsitz SR, et al. Mortality trends after a voluntary checklist-based surgical safety collaborative. Ann Surg 2017;266(6):923–9.
26. Niermeyer S. Global gains after helping babies breathe. Acta Paediatr 2017; 106(10):1550–1.
27. Butz S, editor. Perioperative drill-based crisis management. Cambridge (England): Cambridge University Press; 2016.
28. Hirshey Dirksen SJ, Van Wicklin SA, Mashman DL, et al. Developing effective drills in preparation for a malignant hyperthermia crisis. AORN J 2013;97(3): 329–53.
29. Wang EE. Simulation and adult learning. Dis Mon 2011;57(11):664–78.
30. Ferrari M. The pursuit of excellence through education. Mahwah (NJ): L. Erlbaum Associates; 2002.
31. Issurin VB. Training transfer: scientific background and insights for practical application. Sports Med 2013;43(8):675–94.
32. Zentgraf K, Munzert J, Bischoff M, et al. Simulation during observation of human actions: theories, empirical studies, applications. Vision Res 2011;51(8):827–35.
33. McCoy CE, Sayegh J, Rahman A, et al. Prospective randomized crossover study of telesimulation versus standard simulation for teaching medical students the management of critically ill patients. AEM Educ Train 2017;1(4):287–92.
34. Bong CL, Lee S, Ng ASB, et al. The effects of active (hot-seat) versus observer roles during simulation-based training on stress levels and non-technical performance: a randomized trial. Adv Simul (Lond) 2017;2:7.
35. Lai A, Haligua A, Dylan Bould M, et al. Learning crisis resource management: practicing versus an observational role in simulation training - a randomized controlled trial. Anaesth Crit Care Pain Med 2016;35(4):275–81.
36. Vortman R. Using simulation-based education to improve team communication during a massive transfusion protocol in the OR. AORN J 2020;111(4):393–400.
37. World Telecommunication/ICT Development Report 2010 - MONITORING THE WSIS TARGETS. Available at: http://www.itu.int/ITU-D/ict/publications/wtdr_10/index.html. Accessed February 11, 2019.
38. Mikrogianakis A, Kam A, Silver S, et al. Telesimulation: an innovative and effective tool for teaching novel intraosseous insertion techniques in developing countries. Acad Emerg Med 2011;18(4):420–7.
39. Okrainec A, Henao O, Azzie G. Telesimulation: an effective method for teaching the fundamentals of laparoscopic surgery in resource-restricted countries. Surg Endosc 2010;24(2):417–22.
40. ACLS megacode simulator | ACLS-Algorithms.com. Available at: https://acls-algorithms.com/acls-megacode-simulator/acls-simulator/. Accessed April 10, 2020.

41. Nacca N, Holliday J, Ko PY. Randomized trial of a novel ACLS teaching tool: does it improve student performance? West J Emerg Med 2014;15(7):913–8.
42. Nelson CK, Schwid HA. Screen-based simulation for anesthesiology. Int Anesthesiol Clin 2015;53(4):81–97.
43. American Society of Anesthesiologists and CAE Healthcare Launch Next Generation in Virtual Simulation Training with Anesthesia SimSTAT. American Society of Anesthesiologists. 2019. Available at: https://www.asahq.org/about-asa/newsroom/news-releases/2019/11/american-society-of-anesthesiologists-and-cae-healthcare-launch-next-generation-in-virtual-simulation-training-with-anesthesia-simstat. Accessed March 8, 2020.
44. Drummond D, Hadchouel A, Tesnière A. Serious games for health: three steps forwards. Adv Simul (Lond) 2017;2:3.
45. Wang R, DeMaria S, Goldberg A, et al. A systematic review of serious games in training health care professionals. Simul Healthc 2016;11(1):41–51.
46. Kurenov SN, Cance WW, Noel B, et al. Game-based mass casualty burn training. Stud Health Technol Inform 2009;142:142–4.
47. Rouse C, Bertozzi E, Villafuerte A, et al. 472: Emergency birth!: piloting video game technology as a tool for training critical practices for maternal and neonatal survival among traditional birth attendants. Am J Obstet Gynecol 2014;210(1):S236–7.
48. 3DiTeams - Wikipedia. Available at: https://en.wikipedia.org/wiki/3DiTeams. Accessed December 28, 2018.
49. Honda R, McCoy CE. Teledebriefing in medical simulation. StatPearls. Treasure Island (FL): StatPearls Publishing; 2020.
50. Ahmed R, King Gardner A, Atkinson SS, et al. Teledebriefing: connecting learners to faculty members. Clin Teach 2014;11(4):270–3.
51. Ahmed RA, Atkinson SS, Gable B, et al. Coaching from the sidelines: examining the impact of teledebriefing in simulation-based training. Simul Healthc 2016;11(5):334–9.
52. Brett-Fleegler M, Rudolph J, Eppich W, et al. Debriefing assessment for simulation in healthcare: development and psychometric properties. Simul Healthc 2012;7(5):288–94.
53. Ikeyama T, Shimizu N, Ohta K. Low-cost and ready-to-go remote-facilitated simulation-based learning. Simul Healthc 2012;7(1):35–9.
54. Acton RD, Chipman JG, Lunden M, et al. Unanticipated teaching demands rise with simulation training: strategies for managing faculty workload. J Surg Educ 2015;72(3):522–9.
55. Cheng A, Hunt EA, Donoghue A, et al. Examining pediatric resuscitation education using simulation and scripted debriefing: a multicenter randomized trial. JAMA Pediatr 2013;167(6):528–36.
56. Boet S, Bould MD, Sharma B, et al. Within-team debriefing versus instructor-led debriefing for simulation-based education: a randomized controlled trial. Ann Surg 2013;258(1):53–8.
57. Boese T, Cato M, Gonzalez L, et al. Standards of best practice: simulation standard V: facilitator. Clin Simul Nurs 2013;9(6):S22–5.
58. Blazeck A. Simulation anxiety syndrome: presentation and treatment. Clin Simul Nurs 2011;7(2):e57–60.

Opportunities to Improve the Capacity to Rescue
Intraoperative and Perioperative Tools

Thomas T. Klumpner, MD[a,b,*], Nader N. Massarweh, MD, MPH[c,d,e], Sachin Kheterpal, MD, MBA[a]

KEYWORDS

- Anesthesiology • Perioperative medicine • Postoperative care • Failure to rescue
- Quality improvement • Information technology • Crisis management

KEY POINTS

- Failure to rescue, or the death of a patient after a potentially treatable complication, may be a useful construct to explore variation in health care quality.
- Early recognition and an efficient, coordinated team response to life-threatening complications are essential to prevent failure to rescue.
- Electronic detection algorithms, simulation training, emergency checklists, and a variety of other tools in the perioperative setting may prevent failure to rescue.

INTRODUCTION

Nearly 20 years ago, the Institute of Medicine (IOM) declared that 44,000 to 98,000 Americans die each year as a result of preventable medical errors.[1] The average American has 9 surgical procedures over the course of an 85-year lifespan,[2] and postoperative complications, which occur in approximately 23% of surgeries,[3] are a major source of patient mortality. It is therefore not surprising that close to half of quality measures in the Medicare Quality Payment Program involve a surgical specialty. Although postoperative complications represent a major driver of health care use

[a] Department of Anesthesiology, University of Michigan, 1H247 University Hospital, 1500 East Medical Center Drive, Ann Arbor, MI 48109-5048, USA; [b] Department of Obstetrics and Gynecology, University of Michigan, L4001 Women's Hospital, 1500 East Medical Center Drive, Ann Arbor, MI 48109-0276, USA; [c] Center for Innovations in Quality, Effectiveness and Safety, Michael E DeBakey VAMC, 2002 Holcombe Boulevard, OCL 112, Houston, TX 77030, USA; [d] Michael E DeBakey Department of Surgery, Baylor College of Medicine, Houston, TX, USA; [e] Section of Health Services Research, Department of Medicine, Baylor College of Medicine, Houston, TX, USA
* Corresponding author. Department of Anesthesiology, University of Michigan, 1H247 University Hospital, 1500 East Medical Center Drive, Ann Arbor, MI 48109-5048.
E-mail address: klumpner@med.umich.edu

Anesthesiology Clin 38 (2020) 775–787
https://doi.org/10.1016/j.anclin.2020.08.007
1932-2275/20/© 2020 Elsevier Inc. All rights reserved.
anesthesiology.theclinics.com

and cost,[4] it is unclear whether national quality improvement programs directed at reducing specific postoperative complications have had their intended effect.

A growing body of research suggests the local system's response to a complication is a more important indicator of the quality of care.[5-7] These studies suggest that failure to rescue (FTR), or the death of a patient after a potentially treatable complication, might be a more useful lens through which variation in the quality of care should be examined. FTR acknowledges that complications occur, even when care may have been appropriate, and recognizes the importance of how well complications are managed.[8] In addition, although complications are often associated with patient characteristics, FTR is associated with factors that reflect the setting in which care is delivered.[9-11]

The primary focus of FTR is how the system responds to complications after they occur, with the intent of identifying opportunities to intervene and avert further clinical decline that ends in mortality. Key components of this response include prompt recognition and efficient, coordinated treatment. System factors, including interactions among care team members and institutional safety culture, also play important roles.[9] A recent review provides a good overview of the concept of FTR and explores potentially modifiable factors across the perioperative period.[8]

This narrative review builds on this work by exploring factors and contexts during the intraoperative period, in the postanesthesia care unit (PACU), perioperatively, and after discharge that may represent opportunities to intervene and prevent FTR. It focuses on potential opportunities to improve the response to complications in these unique care settings and discusses tools that may aid in the identification and response to life-threatening complications.

INTRAOPERATIVE FAILURE TO RESCUE

Operating room crises, such as hemorrhage and anaphylaxis, that result in intraoperative death are uncommon events.[12] In one study evaluating 53,718 anesthetics in a Brazilian teaching hospital, 186 perioperative cardiac arrests (94.6% occurring intraoperatively) resulted in 118 deaths (0.2% of all cases).[13] Although not all physiologic insults result in death within the operating room, critical intraoperative events resulting in severe hypotension, severe hypoxemia, and other derangements in homeostasis may still contribute to postoperative mortality. For example, the severity and duration of intraoperative hypotension are associated with 1-year mortality.[14]

Intraoperative critical events that could be associated with a patient's death can unfold rapidly, and the speed with which such an event is recognized and treated affects patient outcome.[15] Intraoperative care requires timely, focused, accurate interpretation of a variety of constantly changing clinical data streams. Because of the complexity of intraoperative care, distractions are common and the chance of errors occurring is high.[16]

Clinical decision support systems (CDSSs) are software products capable of rapidly assimilating a variety of data streams that can potentially aid in making immediate, patient-specific recommendations.[17] Although CDSSs have limitations, these systems are not subject to human error associated with distractions and fatigue. These software systems can direct clinicians' focus to specific life-threatening intraoperative problems as they develop. In doing so, intraoperative CDSSs can improve the recognition of critical events in the operating room. For example, malignant hyperthermia (MH) is a unique, life-threatening adverse reaction that is triggered by certain types of anesthetic agents. Complications increase substantially for every 10-minute delay in treatment.[18] Electronic detection algorithms built into an existing CDSS may improve MH detection. One such system, developed at the Mayo Clinic, decreases time to detect MH crises.[19] Although its effect on MH-associated mortality is unknown, these preliminary results are promising.

Prompt recognition of an evolving intraoperative crisis is an essential first step in preventing FTR. However, equally important is a coordinated, effective response. A failure to recognize and/or act can contribute to intraoperative mortality. As such, finding ways to improve the recognition and response to crises is an important, ongoing area of interest. In one study, 61% of anesthesiologists participating in a simulated ventricular fibrillation arrest failed to follow advanced cardiac life support guidelines; 11% failed to give epinephrine and 6% never used the defibrillator.[20]

As discussed in the Alexander A. Hannenberg'article, "Cognitivde Aids In The Management Of Critical Events," in this issue, emergency checklists may reduce errors that can occur when responding to specific intraoperative crises. Emergency checklists can be built into anesthesia information management systems or CDSSs for easy access (**Fig. 1**).[21] In this manner, CDSSs have the potential to function as both an afferent and efferent arm in the recognition and response to an intraoperative crisis. For example, one system, programmed with institutional glucose management guidelines, has been shown to increase desirable glucose management behavior by recognizing deviation from those guidelines and providing corrective recommendations.[22]

Although studies such as these are promising, it remains unclear whether intraoperative use of a CDSS prevents mortality. One large, single-center, retrospective study evaluating intraoperative use of a CDSS found that, although use of a CDSS was associated with a decrease in hypotension, a decrease in crystalloid administration, and a reduction

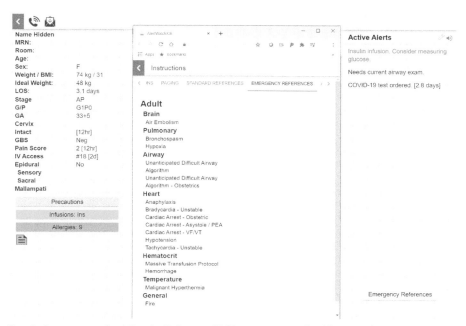

Fig. 1. Emergency checklists built into a CDSS. Emergency checklists can be easily incorporated into real-time CDSSs to allow emergency information to be readily available. Pictured software is AlertWatch OB. Many other CDSSs exist. Please see Refs.[82,83] for further examples. (*Courtesy of* Justin Adams, AlertWatch, Inc., Ann Arbor, MI.)

in cases with median tidal volume in excess of 10 mL/kg, there was no associated decrease in mortality.[23] This finding is surprising given the association of prolonged ventilation with excessive tidal volumes with mortality in the intensive care unit.[24] More studies are needed to determine the effect of intraoperative CDSSs on patient outcome.

Even when a critical event is identified and treatment initiated, the role of teamwork and good communication in preventing FTR cannot be overemphasized. Using an adaptation of crew resource management theory for health care, the Veterans Health Administration introduced intraoperative team training in more than 100 facilities over 3 years.[25] The training intervention encouraged working as a team in the operating room, psychological safety, and use of preoperative and postoperative briefing checklists. Compared with the facilities that were not exposed to the training, there was a near 50% decrease in annual mortality at the facilities that received the team training. There was also a dose-response relationship between amount of team training and surgical mortality reduction: for every quarter of team training, there was a decrease of 0.5 per 1000 procedure-related deaths.[25]

Although mortality within the operating room is rare, many of the intraoperative deaths that do occur may be preventable. Tools such as intraoperative CDSSs, intraoperative emergency checklists, operating team training, and other such interventions that can improve recognition and facilitate a coordinated, appropriate response to intraoperative crises are critical components of any intervention intended to reduce FTR in the operating room.

FAILURE TO RESCUE IN THE POSTANESTHESIA CARE UNIT

According to a prospective survey study published in 1992, as many as 23% of patients in the PACU experience a complication.[26] Although the overall acuity of patient care in the PACU is less than that in the operating room, resources are more constrained. A variable patient census, fixed staffing models, and pressure to accept patients from the operating room may adversely affect staff/patient ratios and potentially reduce the ability to detect a single patient experiencing a rapid deterioration.

More sophisticated staffing algorithms may improve PACU nurse/patient ratios.[27] For example, when applied retrospectively, sophisticated computerized staffing models avoid underestimation of PACU staffing needs better than more conventional methods.[28] Less is understood about adequate physician staffing requirements. Current standards for PACU care require only that a physician be available within the facility.[29] It is not stated whether physician availability should change with a high-acuity and/or a large PACU census. In the emergency department, a unit also typified by variable patient census and acuity, insufficient staffing increases mortality.[30] Sufficient physician and nursing staffing requirements remains an important and poorly understood problem for the PACU that should be further explored.

Even when adequate staff are present, distractions are common and complications may not be easily recognized. As in the operating room, software such as CDSSs may also be leveraged to improve PACU care by improving detection of serious morbidity. Outside of the PACU, CDSSs have been used successfully to improve detection of serious morbidity.[31] However, few such commercial systems exist for PACU use. These tools may be an underused resource to improve PACU care.

One tangible avenue for improvement may exist just before transfer to the PACU. Respiratory complications are the second most frequent PACU complication.[26] Residual neuromuscular blockade (NMB) is likely a direct contributor and may affect as many as 56.5% of patients.[32] Patients that have no reversal of NMB are 5.5 times more likely to require reintubation in the PACU, which is associated with an increased risk of intensive care unit (ICU) admission and death.[33] Standard clinical practice is to antagonize NMB with neostigmine or sugammadex before extubation. Compared with neostigmine and other cholinesterase inhibitors, sugammadex is associated with faster reversal of NMB and fewer adverse events.[34–36] Evidence from a large retrospective observational study also shows that reversal of NMB with sugammadex is associated with a reduced risk of pulmonary complications, including pneumonia and respiratory failure.[37] However, sugammadex is more costly than neostigmine and no clear benefit compared with neostigmine was observed in a large European cohort.[38] Future studies should inform cost-benefit decisions, identify patient populations most likely to benefit from reversal of NMB with sugammadex, and establish opportunities to rescue patients with residual neuromuscular blockade in the PACU.

Patients in the PACU with hypertension or tachycardia have more unplanned ICU admissions and mortality.[39] Whether these cardiovascular events are causative or markers of other underlying conditions is unclear. Nonetheless, this suggests that the PACU may be an important area in which to identify patients at risk of FTR. More needs to be done to better define the complex interplay between PACU events, interventions to improve PACU care, and patient outcome. In efforts to reduce FTR across the continuum of perioperative care, the PACU remains a blind spot.

FAILURE TO RESCUE IN THE PERIOPERATIVE PERIOD

Early recognition of postoperative complications inside and outside of the operating room and a coordinated, effective response are key to preventing patients from progressing to mortality. Early warning systems have the potential to predict transfer to an ICU, in-hospital cardiac arrest, and death before it occurs.[40] These systems are typically based on points allocated to predetermined deviations in vital signs and used to trigger the care team to evaluate the patient's clinical status or to prompt an escalation of care. Some early warning systems have remarkable discriminatory capability. For example, one system, using respiratory rate, peripheral pulse oximetry, use of supplemental oxygen, temperature, systolic blood pressure, heart rate, and level of consciousness, had an area under the receiver operating characteristic curve of 0.894 for prediction of death within 24 hours.[40] Given their potential to improve early recognition of patient deterioration, widespread implementation and use of early warning systems has been recommended.[41]

However, an important piece of data that should be integrated into these point-of-care evaluations and the triggering of a rapid response team is the level of the bedside provider's concern. For example, the so-called nursing worry factor correlates with transfer to the ICU.[42] Although the composition of rapid response teams across hospitals varies greatly, many rapid response teams are nurse led and generally include a nurse with critical care training and a respiratory therapist.[43] Many hospitals implementing rapid response teams have seen a reduction in cardiac arrest and mortality and their widespread implementation has also been endorsed by several health care organizations.[41,44–47]

Improvements in reducing postoperative FTR contributed to a reduction of surgical mortality from 2005 to 2014.[48] In the United States, although many surgical subspecialties have seen a reduction in postoperative mortality,[49,50] one notable exception is maternal mortality, which has progressively increased over the past decade.[51] This increase is in stark contrast to other developed countries, which have seen declines in maternal mortality.[52] It is estimated that as many as 40% of maternal deaths in the United States are preventable, with delayed or inadequate response to clinical warning signs as leading contributory factors.[53,54] As such, maternal mortality provides an excellent representative example to inform a broader discussion around FTR and the preventive interventions discussed to this point.

The National Partnership for Maternal Safety has encouraged hospitals to adopt the Maternal Early Warning Criteria (MEWC), a set of vital sign thresholds for escalation of care, in an effort to reduce delays in the recognition and treatment of maternal morbidity.[55] However, despite the reduction in mortality seen when these systems are combined with rapid response teams, early warning systems are prone to errors in human cognition and heuristic biases. For example, bedside providers must first recognize a change in a patient's condition and be willing to communicate their concerns with other members of the care team. Moreover, although sensitivity is important for any screening tool, a large number of patients that screen positive may limit comprehensive adoption of an early warning system. For example, in a labor and delivery unit with 4600 deliveries per year, one set of vital signs met the MEWC every 9 minutes.[56] Responding to this frequency of aberrant vital signs is impractical.

As such, modifications to the MEWC incorporated into computerized early warning systems that automatically notify providers of a patient's sustained clinical deteriorations are being investigated as a potential avenue to mitigate these limitations.[56] These automated, computerized systems have shown promising early results and have been successful in identifying patients at risk of death in real time outside of labor and delivery.[57,58] On the obstetrics ward, using an automated, computerized system (**Fig. 2**) in conjunction with a nurse-driven maternal early warning system has helped to identify more cases of severe postpartum hemorrhage than either system alone.[31]

As in the management of intraoperative crises, emergency checklists or protocols also improve the response to maternal crises. For example, in postpartum hemorrhage, a leading cause of preventable maternal death,[54,59] adoption of a maternal

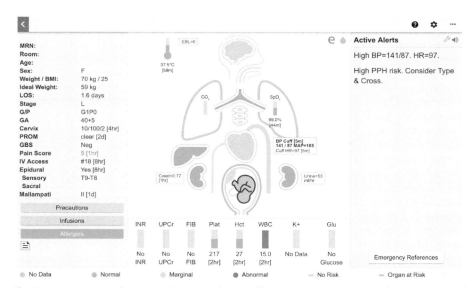

Fig. 2. An automated maternal electronic surveillance system. Automated, computerized surveillance systems have the potential to improve care. Potentially actionable conditions can be easily identified and presented for review, and, if warranted by their severity, paged out to clinical providers. Pictured software is AlertWatch OB. (*Courtesy of* Justin Adams, AlertWatch, Inc., Ann Arbor, MI, AlertWatch, Inc., Ann Arbor, MI.)

hemorrhage protocol improves management.[60] Simulation training may also be an important tool to improve maternal FTR. In 6 rural and urban nonacademic medical centers, simulation training improved time to hemorrhage recognition, time to oxytocin use, time to secondary uterotonic use, and time to performing uterine massage.[61]

Just as postpartum hemorrhage is a leading cause of preventable maternal death, in other specialties specific types of complications may be associated with a higher risk of FTR. For example, following noncardiac surgery, FTR occurs more commonly after acute myocardial infarction and acute renal failure than deep space surgical site infection.[62] Understanding these epidemiologic patterns may lead to more effective methods of arresting the cascade of complications that are thought to follow and may be another useful avenue for improving rescue.

POSTDISCHARGE FAILURE TO RESCUE

For surgical patients, an increasing proportion of their postoperative recovery after inpatient procedures is shifting from the hospital to the outpatient setting. For example, procedures once associated with a postoperative inpatient stay, such as total knee arthroplasty, are now routinely performed in the ambulatory surgical setting. Furthermore, the average length of stay for surgical admissions has decreased significantly over the past 2 decades.[63] This shift in how perioperative care is provided, along with the fact that it is unclear that all types of complications and readmissions are predictable, preventable, and/or avoidable,[64] brings with it unique challenges for the recognition and treatment of postoperative complications. Nearly one-third of postoperative complications occur after discharge.[3] Therefore, because one of the most critical factors affecting FTR is early recognition, this prompts the question of how best to identify and address evolving complications in postoperative patients in the outpatient setting? After discharge, patients and their families are typically the first line of recognition for an evolving complication. As such, a well-designed approach to educating patients and their families on postoperative care, the most significant procedure-related complications, as well as the early warning signs is essential and should begin at the initial consultation. To avoid overwhelming the patient, ideally this education should continue throughout the preoperative period.[65] In addition, at discharge the patients and their families should be provided with reliable contact information for providers who can advise them during and after regular clinic hours.

Patients who live remotely relative to the hospital where their operation is performed present an additional, unique challenge. Postoperative care continuity has an important association with patient outcomes: patients readmitted to the same hospital where their operation was performed and who receive care from the same surgical team involved in their initial postoperative care have a significantly lower risk of death.[66] When patients are having a complication and need immediate care from a hospital in their local community, resources available at the hospital where the operation was performed may not be available (eg, interventional radiology, advanced endoscopy) and the local providers may not have the knowledge or expertise to appropriately recognize, diagnose, and treat the issue. Remote, postdischarge consultation could address the need for early recognition of a developing complication and could aid in the prompt treatment or transfer of the patient.

Mobile health and telemedicine technology represents existing tools that could be leveraged to at least partially address these issues. In-phone cameras are now available on virtually every type of mobile phone and can be used by patients to send images or videos to clinical care teams in any location.[67–71] As patients spend less time in the hospital recovering after inpatient surgical procedures, these tools can be leveraged to ensure patients who live at a distance from the clinical care team can remain in contact and that their postoperative recovery is progressing appropriately. For example, a smartphone can be used as an accelerometer to capture information about a patient's baseline, preoperative activity to create a digital phenotype.[72] This baseline information can then be compared with postoperative activity to allow the care team to not only ensure the patient is appropriately progressing toward recovery benchmarks but also to serve as a potential early warning of an evolving complication in patients who are not achieving expected levels of activity.[73]

An additional issue to consider is the prescription and use of opioids in postoperative patients. There is substantial variation in the amounts of opioids prescribed postoperatively to patients, and opioid overdose accounts for more than 30,000 deaths annually.[74–76] Most states have implemented prescription drug monitoring programs as a centralized effort to provide clinicians with real-time information about patients' prescribing histories at the point of care. However, the effectiveness of these types of programs at modifying opioid prescribing practices remains unclear.[77] It is therefore imperative that clinical care teams be constantly mindful that they are adequately addressing the postoperative pain needs of their surgical patients in a responsible manner. At present, there is little consensus and/or guidance regarding the appropriate type and amount of opioids that should be prescribed in postoperative patients.[78] Although procedure-specific, multidisciplinary pain management guidelines and recommendations have been proposed, until such guidelines are developed, accepted, and implemented for all procedures, surgical care teams should make efforts to maximize the use of nonopioid pain medications when possible and prescribe the lowest effective doses as well as dispensing the minimum number thought to be needed.[79] If patients indicate that they are having continued and/or increasing pain or have a longer than expected requirement for pain medication, this should prompt an evaluation and diagnostic studies (as indicated) to investigate evolving or existing complications as a possible cause.

SUMMARY

Between 1948 and 1952, the number of deaths attributable to anesthesia in the United States was 1 in 1560 (1 in 370 if muscle relaxant was used as part of the anesthetic).[80] As new anesthetic techniques, training, and an increasing emphasis on safety has transformed the specialty of anesthesiology, the risk of death from anesthesia has declined significantly. Data from 1999 to 2005 estimate that the risk of mortality from anesthesia for surgical inpatients is now 1 in 120,000.[81] A careful analysis of workflow, tools, and nearly all aspects of anesthetic care helped make this possible. However, the work is not done. Many perioperative deaths are likely still preventable. CDSSs, simulation, emergency checklists, early warning systems, improved patient education, mobile telehealth applications, and other tools to improve recognition and response to perioperative complications may further reduce FTR.

CLINICS CARE POINTS

- Point of care clinical decision support systems may reduce time to recognize critical events.
- Emergency checklists and protocols improve response to severe morbidity.
- Mobile health and telemedicine have the potential to improve recognition of post-discharge complications.

DISCLOSURE

This article is based on work supported by the US Department of Veterans Affairs Health Services Research and Development Service of the VA Office of Research and Development Merit Review (I01 HX002447, N.N. Massarweh) and the Center for Innovations in Quality, Effectiveness and Safety (CIN [Center of Innovation] 13-413, N.N.M.). The authors have no conflicts of interest to disclose.

REFERENCES

1. Institute of Medicine & Committee on Quality of Health Care in America. To err is human: building a safer health system. Washington, DC: National Academies Press; 2000.
2. Lee PHU, Gawande AA. The number of surgical procedures in an American lifetime in 3 states. J Am Coll Surg Vol 2008;207:S75.
3. Morris MS, Deierhoi RJ, Richman JS, et al. The relationship between timing of surgical complications and hospital readmission. JAMA Surg 2014;149(4):348–54.
4. Birkmeyer JD, Gust C, Dimick JB, et al. Hospital quality and the cost of inpatient surgery in the United States. Ann Surg 2012;255(1):1–5.
5. Silber JH, Williams SV, Krakauer H, et al. Hospital and patient characteristics associated with death after surgery. A study of adverse occurrence and failure to rescue. Med Care 1992;30(7):615–29.
6. Ghaferi AA, Birkmeyer JD, Dimick JB. Variation in hospital mortality associated with inpatient surgery. N Engl J Med 2009;361(14):1368–75.
7. Massarweh NN, Anaya DA, Kougias P, et al. Variation and Impact of Multiple Complications on Failure to Rescue After Inpatient Surgery. Ann Surg 2017; 266(1):59–65.
8. Portuondo JI, Shah SR, Singh H, et al. Failure to Rescue as a Surgical Quality Indicator: Current Concepts and Future Directions for Improving Surgical Outcomes. Anesthesiology 2019;131(2):426–37.
9. Ghaferi AA, Dimick JB. Importance of teamwork, communication and culture on failure-to-rescue in the elderly. Br J Surg 2016;103(2):e47–51.
10. Rosero EB, Joshi GP, Minhajuddin A, et al. Effects of hospital safety-net burden and hospital volume on failure to rescue after open abdominal aortic surgery. J Vasc Surg 2017;66(2):404–12.
11. Pandit V, Jehan F, Zeeshan M, et al. Failure to Rescue in Postoperative Patients With Colon Cancer: Time to Rethink Where You Get Surgery. J Surg Res 2019; 234:1–6.
12. Bainbridge D, Martin J, Arango M, et al, Evidence-based Peri-operative Clinical Outcomes Research (EPiCOR) Group. Perioperative and anaesthetic-related mortality in developed and developing countries: a systematic review and meta-analysis. Lancet 2012;380(9847):1075–81.
13. Braz LG, Módolo NS, do Nascimento P, et al. Perioperative cardiac arrest: a study of 53,718 anaesthetics over 9 yr from a Brazilian teaching hospital. Br J Anaesth 2006;96(5):569–75.
14. Bijker JB, van Klei WA, Vergouwe Y, et al. Intraoperative hypotension and 1-year mortality after noncardiac surgery. Anesthesiology 2009;111(6):1217–26.
15. Dutton RP, Lee LA, Stephens LS, et al. Massive hemorrhage: a report from the anesthesia closed claims project. Anesthesiology 2014;121(3):450–8.
16. Sevdalis N, Undre S, McDermott J, et al. Impact of intraoperative distractions on patient safety: a prospective descriptive study using validated instruments. World J Surg 2014;38(4):751–8.

17. Sim I, Gorman P, Greenes RA, et al. Clinical decision support systems for the practice of evidence-based medicine. J Am Med Inform Assoc 2001;8(6): 527–34.

18. Riazi S, Larach MG, Hu C, et al. Malignant hyperthermia in Canada: characteristics of index anesthetics in 129 malignant hyperthermia susceptible probands. Anesth Analg 2014;118(2):381–7.

19. Gleich SJ, Strupp K, Wilder RT, et al. An automated real-time method for the detection of patients at risk for malignant hyperthermia. Paediatr Anaesth 2016; 26(9):876–82.

20. Kurrek MM, Devitt JH, Cohen M. Cardiac arrest in the OR: how are our ACLS skills? Can J Anaesth 1998;45(2):130–2.

21. Tremper KK, Mace JJ, Gombert JM, et al. Design of a Novel Multifunction Decision Support Display for Anesthesia Care: AlertWatch® OR. BMC Anesthesiol 2018;18(1):16.

22. Sathishkumar S, Lai M, Picton P, et al. Behavioral Modification of Intraoperative Hyperglycemia Management with a Novel Real-time Audiovisual Monitor. Anesthesiology 2015;123(1):29–37.

23. Kheterpal S, Shanks A, Tremper KK. Impact of a Novel Multiparameter Decision Support System on Intraoperative Processes of Care and Postoperative Outcomes. Anesthesiology 2018;128(2):272–82.

24. Sjoding MW, Gong MN, Haas CF, et al. Evaluating Delivery of Low Tidal Volume Ventilation in Six ICUs Using Electronic Health Record Data. Crit Care Med 2019; 47(1):56–61.

25. Neily J, Mills PD, Young-Xu Y, et al. Association between implementation of a medical team training program and surgical mortality. JAMA 2010;304(15): 1693–700.

26. Hines R, Barash PG, Watrous G, et al. Complications occurring in the postanesthesia care unit: a survey. Anesth Analg 1992;74(4):503–9.

27. Dexter F, Wachtel RE, Epstein RH. Impact of average patient acuity on staffing of the phase I PACU. J Perianesth Nurs 2006;21(5):303–10.

28. Siddiqui S, Morse E, Levin S. Evaluating nurse staffing levels in perianesthesia care units using discrete event simulation., vol. 7. Oxfordshire (UK): Taylor & Francis; 2017. p. 215–23. IISE Transactions on Healthcare Systems Engineering.

29. Committee on Standards and Practice Parameters. Standards for Postanesthesia Care. American Society of Anesthesiologists. 2019. Available at: https://www.asahq.org/standards-and-guidelines/standards-for-postanesthesia-care. Accessed April 30, 2020.

30. Morley C, Unwin M, Peterson GM, et al. Emergency department crowding: A systematic review of causes, consequences and solutions. PLoS One 2018;13(8): e0203316.

31. Klumpner TT, Kountanis JA, Meyer SR, et al. Use of a Novel Electronic Maternal Surveillance System and the Maternal Early Warning Criteria to Detect Severe Postpartum Hemorrhage. Anesth Analg 2020. https://doi.org/10.1213/ANE.0000000000004605.

32. Fortier L-P, McKeen D, Turner K, et al. The RECITE Study: A Canadian Prospective, Multicenter Study of the Incidence and Severity of Residual Neuromuscular Blockade. Anesth Analg 2015;121(2):366–72.

33. Belcher AW, Leung S, Cohen B, et al. Incidence of complications in the postanesthesia care unit and associated healthcare utilization in patients undergoing non-cardiac surgery requiring neuromuscular blockade 2005-2013: A single center study. J Clin Anesth 2017;43:33–8.

34. Hristovska A-M, Duch P, Allingstrup M, et al. Efficacy and safety of sugammadex versus neostigmine in reversing neuromuscular blockade in adults. Cochrane Database Syst Rev 2017;(8):CD012763.

35. Sacan O, White PF, Tufanogullari B, et al. Sugammadex reversal of rocuronium-induced neuromuscular blockade: a comparison with neostigmine-glycopyrrolate and edrophonium-atropine. Anesth Analg 2007;104(3):569–74.

36. An J, Lee JH, Kim E, et al. Comparison of sugammadex and pyridostigmine bromide for reversal of rocuronium-induced neuromuscular blockade in short-term pediatric surgery: A prospective randomized study. Medicine (Baltimore) 2020; 99(7):e19130.

37. Kheterpal S, Vaughn MT, Dubovoy TZ, et al. Sugammadex versus Neostigmine for Reversal of Neuromuscular Blockade and Postoperative Pulmonary Complications (STRONGER): A Multicenter Matched Cohort Analysis. Anesthesiology 2020;132(6):1371–81.

38. Kirmeier E, Eriksson LI, Lewald H, et al. Post-anaesthesia pulmonary complications after use of muscle relaxants (POPULAR): a multicentre, prospective observational study. Lancet Respir Med 2019;7(2):129–40.

39. Rose DK, Cohen MM, DeBoer DP. Cardiovascular events in the postanesthesia care unit: contribution of risk factors. Anesthesiology 1996;84(4):772–81.

40. Smith GB, Prytherch DR, Meredith P, et al. The ability of the National Early Warning Score (NEWS) to discriminate patients at risk of early cardiac arrest, unanticipated intensive care unit admission, and death. Resuscitation 2013;84(4): 465–70.

41. Armitage M, Eddleston J, Stokes T, Guideline Development Group at the NICE. Recognising and responding to acute illness in adults in hospital: summary of NICE guidance. BMJ 2007;335(7613):258–9.

42. Romero-Brufau S, Gaines K, Nicolas CT, et al. The fifth vital sign? Nurse worry predicts inpatient deterioration within 24 hours. JAMIA Open 2019;2(4):465.

43. Stolldorf DP, Jones CB. Deployment of rapid response teams by 31 hospitals in a statewide collaborative. Jt Comm J Qual Patient Saf 2015;41(4):186–91.

44. Buist MD, Moore GE, Bernard SA, et al. Effects of a medical emergency team on reduction of incidence of and mortality from unexpected cardiac arrests in hospital: preliminary study. BMJ 2002;324(7334):387–90.

45. Bellomo R, Goldsmith D, Uchino S, et al. A prospective before-and-after trial of a medical emergency team. Med J Aust 2003;179(6):283–7.

46. Santamaria J, Tobin A, Holmes J. Changing cardiac arrest and hospital mortality rates through a medical emergency team takes time and constant review. Crit Care Med 2010;38(2):445–50.

47. Berwick DM, Calkins DR, McCannon CJ, et al. The 100,000 lives campaign: setting a goal and a deadline for improving health care quality. JAMA 2006; 295(3):324–7.

48. Fry BT, Smith ME, Thumma JR, et al. Ten-year Trends in Surgical Mortality, Complications, and Failure to Rescue in Medicare Beneficiaries. Ann Surg 2019. https://doi.org/10.1097/SLA.0000000000003193.

49. Cohen ME, Liu Y, Ko CY, et al. Improved Surgical Outcomes for ACS NSQIP Hospitals Over Time: Evaluation of Hospital Cohorts With up to 8 Years of Participation. Ann Surg 2016;263(2):267–73.

50. Liu JB, Berian JR, Liu Y, et al. Procedure-Specific Trends in Surgical Outcomes. J Am Coll Surg 2018;226(1):30–6.e4.

51. MacDorman MF, Declercq E, Cabral H, et al. Recent Increases in the U.S. Maternal Mortality Rate: Disentangling Trends From Measurement Issues. Obstet Gynecol 2016;128(3):447–55.
52. GBD 2015 Maternal Mortality Collaborators, Kassebaum NJ, Barber RM, Bhutta ZA, et al. Global, regional, and national levels of maternal mortality, 1990–2015: a systematic analysis for the Global Burden of Disease Study 2015. Lancet 2016;388:1775–812.
53. Mitchell C, Lawton E, Morton C, et al. California Pregnancy-Associated Mortality Review: mixed methods approach for improved case identification, cause of death analyses and translation of findings. Matern Child Health J 2014;18(3):518–26.
54. Main EK, McCain CL, Morton CH, et al. Pregnancy-related mortality in California: causes, characteristics, and improvement opportunities. Obstet Gynecol 2015;125(4):938–47.
55. Mhyre JM, D'Oria R, Hameed AB, et al. The maternal early warning criteria: a proposal from the national partnership for maternal safety. Obstet Gynecol 2014;124:782–6.
56. Klumpner TT, Kountanis JA, Langen ES, et al. Use of a novel electronic maternal surveillance system to generate automated alerts on the labor and delivery unit. BMC Anesthesiol 2018;18(1):78.
57. Finlay GD, Rothman MJ, Smith RA. Measuring the modified early warning score and the Rothman index: advantages of utilizing the electronic medical record in an early warning system. J Hosp Med 2014;9(2):116–9.
58. Ye C, Wang O, Liu M, et al. A Real-Time Early Warning System for Monitoring Inpatient Mortality Risk: Prospective Study Using Electronic Medical Record Data. J Med Internet Res 2019;21(7):e13719.
59. Pregnancy Mortality Surveillance System. Centers for Disease Control and Prevention. 2019. Available at: https://www.cdc.gov/reproductivehealth/maternalinfanthealth/pregnancy-mortality-surveillance-system.htm. Accessed April 30, 2020.
60. Shields LE, Wiesner S, Fulton J, et al. Comprehensive maternal hemorrhage protocols reduce the use of blood products and improve patient safety. Am J Obstet Gynecol 2015;212(3):272–80.
61. Marshall NE, Vanderhoeven J, Eden KB, et al. Impact of simulation and team training on postpartum hemorrhage management in non-academic centers. J Matern Fetal Neonatal Med 2015;28(5):495–9.
62. Wakeam E, Hyder JA, Jiang W, et al. Risk and patterns of secondary complications in surgical inpatients. JAMA Surg 2015;150(1):65–73.
63. Nazzani S, Preisser F, Mazzone E, et al. In-hospital length of stay after major surgical oncological procedures. Eur J Surg Oncol 2018;44(7):969–74.
64. van Galen LS, Vedder D, Boeije T, et al. Different Perspectives on Predictability and Preventability of Surgical Readmissions. J Surg Res 2019;237:95–105.
65. Smith AB, Mueller D, Garren B, et al. Using qualitative research to reduce readmissions and optimize perioperative cystectomy care. Cancer 2019;125(20):3545–53.
66. Brooke BS, Goodney PP, Kraiss LW, et al. Readmission destination and risk of mortality after major surgery: an observational cohort study. Lancet 2015;386(9996):884–95.
67. Pérez F, Montón E, Nodal MJ, et al. Evaluation of a mobile health system for supporting postoperative patients following day surgery. J Telemed Telecare 2006;12(Suppl 1):41–3.

68. Gunter R, Fernandes-Taylor S, Mahnke A, et al. Evaluating Patient Usability of an Image-Based Mobile Health Platform for Postoperative Wound Monitoring. JMIR Mhealth Uhealth 2016;4(3):e113.
69. Gunter RL, Chouinard S, Fernandes-Taylor S, et al. Current Use of Telemedicine for Post-Discharge Surgical Care: A Systematic Review. J Am Coll Surg 2016; 222(5):915–27.
70. Williams AM, Bhatti UF, Alam HB, et al. The role of telemedicine in postoperative care. Mhealth 2018;4:11.
71. Gunter RL, Fernandes-Taylor S, Rahman S, et al. Feasibility of an Image-Based Mobile Health Protocol for Postoperative Wound Monitoring. J Am Coll Surg 2018;226(3):277–86.
72. Panda N, Solsky I, Haynes AB. Redefining shared decision-making in the digital era. Eur J Surg Oncol 2019;45(12):2287–8.
73. Panda N, Solsky I, Huang EJ, et al. Using Smartphones to Capture Novel Recovery Metrics After Cancer Surgery. JAMA Surg 2019;155(2):1–7.
74. Hill MV, McMahon ML, Stucke RS, et al. Wide Variation and Excessive Dosage of Opioid Prescriptions for Common General Surgical Procedures. Ann Surg 2017; 265(4):709–14.
75. Thiels CA, Anderson SS, Ubl DS, et al. Wide Variation and Overprescription of Opioids After Elective Surgery. Ann Surg 2017;266(4):564–73.
76. Rudd RA, Seth P, David F, et al. Increases in Drug and Opioid-Involved Overdose Deaths - United States, 2010-2015. MMWR Morb Mortal Wkly Rep 2016;65(5051): 1445–52.
77. Lin H-C, Wang Z, Boyd C, et al. Associations between statewide prescription drug monitoring program (PDMP) requirement and physician patterns of prescribing opioid analgesics for patients with non-cancer chronic pain. Addict Behav 2018;76:348–54.
78. Zhang DDQ, Dossa F, Arora A, et al. Recommendations for the Prescription of Opioids at Discharge After Abdominopelvic Surgery: A Systematic Review. JAMA Surg 2020. https://doi.org/10.1001/jamasurg.2019.5875.
79. Overton HN, Hanna MN, Bruhn WE, et al. Opioid-Prescribing Guidelines for Common Surgical Procedures: An Expert Panel Consensus. J Am Coll Surg 2018; 227(4):411–8.
80. Beecher HK, Todd DP. A study of the deaths associated with anesthesia and surgery: based on a study of 599, 548 anesthesias in ten institutions 1948-1952, inclusive. Ann Surg 1954;140(1):2–35.
81. Li G, Warner M, Lang BH, et al. Epidemiology of Anesthesia-related Mortality in the United States, 1999–2005. Anesthesiology 2009;110(4):759–65.
82. Nair BG, Gabel E, Hofer I, et al. Intraoperative Clinical Decision Support for Anesthesia. Anesth Analg 2017;124(2):603–17.
83. Simpao AF, Tan JM, Lingappan AM, et al. A systematic review of near real-time and point-of-care clinical decision support in anesthesia information management systems. J Clin Monit Comput 2017;31:885–94.

Cognitive Aids in the Management of Critical Events

Alexander A. Hannenberg, MD[a,b,*]

KEYWORDS

- Checklists • Critical events • Operating room

KEY POINTS

- Cognitive aids can augment clinician training and memory to improve management of critical events.
- Acceptance of these tools in practice requires a cultural change that recognizes clinicians' fallibility, especially under stress.
- Implementation of checklists and emergency manuals is a multifaceted and cross-professional process that should be carefully planned.

Operating room critical events share many of the characteristics of an aircraft engine failure: they threaten severe consequences and are exceedingly rare, meaning that no clinician (or pilot) is likely to have recent experience in their management. They induce significant psychological stress, the deleterious effect of which on memory and performance is discussed in detail in Barbara K. Burian and R. Key Dismukes' article, "Why We Fail to Rescue During Critical Events," in this issue. In both the operating room and the cockpit, the synergy of drills with simulated crises and availability of a purpose-designed reference tool make both of these essential elements of preparedness. The role of simulated practice drills is addressed specifically in Amanda R. Burden's article, "High-Fidelity Simulation Education and Crisis Resource Management"; and Megan Delisle and Alexander A. Hannenberg's article, "Alternatives to High-Fidelity Simulation," in this issue and also throughout the articles in this volume. This article focuses on the role of cognitive aids, such as crisis checklists or emergency manuals (terms that are used interchangeably in this article and in the literature), in supporting clinicians in optimizing the management and outcomes of critical events.

Conflict of interest: The author declares no conflict of interest and that this work received no external funding.
[a] Ariadne Labs, 401 Park Drive 3-West, Boston, MA 02215, USA; [b] Tufts University School of Medicine, Boston, MA, USA
* Ariadne Labs, 401 Park Drive 3-West, Boston, MA 02215.
E-mail address: ahannenberg@ariadnelabs.org

BACKGROUND

Checklists were introduced into aviation in the 1930s as aircraft systems became more complex and pilots recognized the risk of cognitive overload in flying them. The pivotal moment came when a new military aircraft crashed during its demonstration flight in 1935 and the commission studying the event recommended the use of aviation checklists.[1] They have been standard practice in civilian and commercial aviation ever since, and also adopted in several other high-reliability organizations. Checklists are used to support routine activities and also nonroutine or emergency responses; this is true in medicine and elsewhere. In the operating room, checklists have been used to support the anesthesia machine checkout[2](routine) and management of malignant hyperthermia (nonroutine) for decades.[3] The concept of emergency checklists for the operating room was promoted as early as 1924 by the Philadelphia surgeon W. Wayne Babock,[4] whose recommendation was entirely overlooked at the time. Meaningful momentum for the use of checklists in health care was gained 80 years later with the validation of the World Health Organization (WHO) Safe Surgery Checklist[5] and the Central Line Insertion Checklist.[6] The WHO Safe Surgery Checklist is now used in nearly 90% of operating rooms in high-income countries.[7]

Although operating room crisis checklists have many valuable uses, they are principally designed for real-time management of critical events. They are distinct in their content and design from textbooks, guidelines, or manuals. The content generally has its basis in such sources, but it is highly distilled and content meets inclusion criteria such as the likelihood of omission, consequences of omission, and susceptibility to improvement by inclusion in a checklist.[8] Some checklist content may exist to explicitly provoke team discussion. The layout (fonts, space, color, graphics, word count) is optimized for rapid reference under stress. These principles are outlined in "A Checklist for Checklists"[9] which was developed in collaboration with aviation checklist experts. Familiarity with these design principles is important for end users to allow them to modify and customize the checklists while preserving the key design qualities. A recent simulation-based comparison of the effectiveness of linear checklist design and branched logic design suggested that team performance was superior when using a linear checklist design.[10] Regardless of the specific checklist chosen, users must become familiar with the design features, such as the significance of colors used and the expected location and appearance of different types of information, such as drug doses and differential diagnosis prompts. This familiarity is essential for both effective use and for locally driven modifications. Users cannot be expected to understand layout and content on their first exposure to the tools, and this is one of the myriad reasons to introduce them into practice with a carefully designed training program.

EXPERIENCE

For operating room teams, cognitive aids for critical events have appeared from numerous sources over the past several decades. The best-known crisis checklists are compendia that address several critical events. These compendia have been produced by the Stanford Anesthesia Cognitive Aid Group,[11] Ariadne Labs at the Harvard T.H. Chan School of Public Health and Brigham and Women's Hospital,[12] and the Society for Pediatric Anesthesia (SPA).[13] Although these are more similar than different, the scope of the events addressed, design, and format (paper or electronic) differ. There have been translations of these tools into Chinese, Spanish and other languages. These 3 compendia and some others have been made available without charge by their developers and have been downloaded more than 200,000 times worldwide. Over the years, there have been other crisis checklist compendia created and individual checklists developed for specific operating room emergencies, a sample of which are listed in **Table 1**. The Emergency Manuals Implementation Collaborative Web site contains links to many of them.[14]

EVIDENCE

The rarity and unpredictability of the events addressed by these tools has limited the study of their impact on patient care to simulated operating room emergencies. Weinger estimated that an assessment of the impact of cognitive aids on patient outcomes would require study of 1.6 million patients over 3 years.[30] The several major simulation studies of cognitive aids have been consistent in their findings of favorable

Table 1
Selected operating room critical event cognitive aids

Checklist	Source	Type	Notes
Neuroanesthetic emergency	Society for Neuroscience in Anesthesiology and Critical Care Education Committee[15]	Event specific	—
Intraoperative neuromonitoring changes	Ziewacz[16]; Vitale[17]	Event specific	—
Local anesthetic systemic toxicity	American Society of Regional Anesthesia and Pain[18]	Event specific	—
Mass casualty	American Society of Anesthesiologists[19]	Event specific	Members-only access
Robotic surgery hemorrhage	Nepple et al[20]	Event specific	—
Neonatal resuscitation	Katheria et al[21]	Event specific	—
Trauma anesthesia	Tobin et al[22]	Event specific	—
Malignant hyperthermia protocol	Malignant Hyperthermia Association of the United States[23]	Event specific	—
Cardiac surgery emergencies	2018 IEEE Conference on Cognitive and Computational Aspects of Situation Management[24]	Event specific	—
Quick Reference Handbook	Association of Anaesthetists of Great Britain and Ireland[25]	Compendium	—
Stanford OB Anesthesia Emergency Manual	Stanford Cognitive Aids in Medicine Group[26]	Compendium	—
Anaesthetic Crisis Manual	Borshoff[27]	Compendium	For purchase
Crisis Management in Anesthesiology	Gaba et al[28]	Compendium	For purchase
A Visual Guide to Crisis Management	Chu & Fuller[29]	Compendium	For purchase

Abbreviation: IEEE, Institute of Electrical and Electronics Engineers; OB, obstetric.
Data from Refs.[15–29]

impact on completeness and accuracy of patient care. Arriaga and colleagues'[31] simulation study of crisis checklists in the *New England Journal of Medicine* was highly influential. Multidisciplinary teams from both academic and community facilities were exposed to high-fidelity simulation of multiple critical events and alternately managed them with the use of a crisis checklist and without. They were scored against a matrix of essential management steps and, when using checklists, the operating room teams were 75% less likely to omit critical steps. The participants had very favorable ratings of the checklists after using them in the simulation trial. Similarly, Neal and colleagues[32] studied trainees' management of a simulated local anesthetic systemic toxicity (LAST) reaction with and without the American Society of Regional Anesthesia LAST checklist and found that use of the checklist doubled the number of key management steps completed. At Stanford, Harrison and colleagues[33] found that the frequency of cognitive aid use correlated closely with a score reflecting the completeness of management in a simulated malignant hyperthermia event. Malignant hyperthermia simulations were also the setting for a more recent evaluation of checklist impact, with similarly positive findings on both technical and nontechnical performance.[34] Users frequently report that, even when the checklist confirms that all needed steps were being addressed, the benefits of this reassurance were valuable in focusing the team on the care of the patient and relieving the cognitive stress of pondering missing steps.

EFFECTIVE USE

Use of cognitive aids during critical events does not replace clinical judgment and decision making by the user, beginning with the real-time determination that reference to a checklist is warranted. There are clearly some operating room critical events that will be quickly resolved without need for reference to a checklist, just as is the case with aviation emergencies. For example, transient bradycardia is most often treated successfully with a single intravenous dose of an anticholinergic. When this, or perhaps a familiar second-line therapy, does not produce the desired response, a cognitive aid can lay out other, less commonly used options and support the application of these options with information not otherwise readily at hand, such as constitution of intravenous drips, dosages of uncommon medications, and operation instructions for pacemakers. In this scenario, the anesthesia providers may initially refer to the aid in isolation. Understanding the trigger for checklist use is a component of learning the effective application of these tools through experience or, more realistically, simulation. Recognition that there are management steps that must be immediately implemented from memory is an important lesson to emphasize during introduction of the tools. Users will be more apt to accept the concept of cognitive aids if it is made clear that, in the case of an operating room fire, for example, it is expected that steps will be taken before consulting the checklists.

In other, more complex critical events, such as malignant hyperthermia or uncontrolled hemorrhage, that demand engagement from the larger perioperative team, the cognitive aid is of value to all. Particularly in such events, engaging a team member in the task of reading the checklist aloud serves multiple purposes.[35] It unburdens the crisis manager from the task, readily fosters a shared mental model among members of the team, and facilitates assignment of specific tasks. These features can promote effective teamwork, whose absence is a major contributor to adverse outcomes.[36,37] The value of assigning a nonanesthetist reader when these aids are used argues for a multidisciplinary introduction and training to establish buy-in, familiarity, and readiness to accept the reader role when needed.

Engagement of the entire operating room team in the introduction of checklists has the additional effect of increasing the likelihood that the tool will be used when needed. Use of an available cognitive aid when needed during a critical event is not to be taken for granted. It is surprising how frequently clinicians who know that the aid is readily available during a crisis do not avail themselves of the tool,[38] thus the importance of a strategy specifically designed to maximize appropriate use. Optimal deployment includes strategic, highly visible placement of the manual, not only for the anesthesia team but often for an additional copy for the circulating nurse. The importance of multidisciplinary introduction and training on the use of the manual includes enabling those other than the anesthesia staff to trigger its use by making the entire surgical team comfortable with the manual and each other. Creating this redundancy is a countermeasure to the risk of any individual failing to use the tool when it could benefit the patient. Recognizing issues of professional hierarchy in training is essential to neutralize the barrier to sharing responsibility for triggering checklist use, as well as supporting effective teamwork more broadly.

As noted, the benefits of the use of cognitive aids for critical events have been reproducibly demonstrated, but, like nearly any intervention in health care, they have risks. At the 2015 Anesthesia Patient Safety Consensus Conference on this subject,[30] Daniel Raemer, a pioneer in health care simulation, discussed several pitfalls, many observed in crisis resource management simulation training in which cognitive aids were used by the participants. An appreciation of these pitfalls drives a deep appreciation of the need for user training for effective and safe use of cognitive aids. Raemer provided several illustrative examples (Raemer D. Emergency Manuals – Pitfalls and Risks. Presented at the: Anesthesia Patient Safety Foundation Consensus Conference; September 15, 2015; Scottsdale AZ. Personal communication.).

Paradoxically, although crisis resource management training emphasizes avoidance of fixation errors, the selection of a particular crisis checklist can promote such errors. When clinicians encounter intraoperative bronchospasm and select a checklist for anaphylaxis, it seems to make them less likely to consider another cause of the bronchospasm. Training checklist users to recognize the difference between a symptom-oriented checklist (eg, hypotension) and a diagnosis-oriented checklist (eg, anaphylaxis) is a key learning objective. Even among diagnosis-oriented checklists, a propensity to fixation is a risk: consider the overlap and diagnostic uncertainty with the possibilities of anaphylaxis and transfusion reaction: choosing a checklist for one can cause clinicians to ignore the other possibility. Checklist users must be trained to expect the coexistence of multiple critical events, such as arrhythmia, hypotension, and hypoxemia. This example clearly underscores the inescapable importance of clinical judgment even with cognitive aids at hand. The author has previously commented on the value of the reader role in the use of checklists, but even this poses a risk. Especially when both reader and manager are physicians, there is a risk of the reader role impinging on the event manager role, potentially compromising the team dynamic.

Very few of the hazards identified by Raemer will be evident to naive users picking up the checklist without an orientation to the elements of safe and effective use. Champions and implementers have a responsibility to address these issues to achieve their goal of improving care: primum non nocere. As with any other clinical tool, the rationale for training in the use of checklists should be evident.

TRAINING

The goals of training are first and foremost to familiarize and socialize the use of these tools. Their use is a clear statement recognizing fallibility, which is a cultural change and represents a departure from a deeply ingrained characteristic of professionalism. At the same time, it is a commitment to putting excellence above pride. Training and implementation are designed to promote these values across the team and institution. For most clinicians, cognitive aids are a new facet in the management of critical events and building acceptance of the concept is a prerequisite for effective use. However, if a clinician's first exposure to the tools is in the midst of an operating room emergency, there is a dramatically diminished likelihood of the checklist improving care.

As adult learners, checklist users derive vastly more benefit from experiential learning than didactic instruction,[39] which makes simulation training, where available, an obvious choice as a platform for achieving the learning objectives discussed. The focus on critical events in crisis resource management simulation curricula makes concurrent training on cognitive aids naturally synergistic. A model of simulation training with multiple advantages is in situ simulation, conducted in an actual patient care setting such as an unscheduled operating room.[40] This approach additionally offers an opportunity to stress test existing systems and resources and identify latent defects.[41] Its technology requirements are minimal and these sessions can be adapted to fit the time constraints of the facility. What in-situ simulation requires, like nearly all variants of simulation-based education, is a simulation educator who is capable of designing the simulation scenario, facilitating it, and leading the debriefing of the participants to safely capture maximum learning from the experience. The scarcity of such individuals outside of academic medical centers represents a challenge for implementers of these tools and others.[42] These matters are more fully discussed in Megan Delisle and Alexander A. Hannenberg's article, "Alternatives to High-Fidelity Simulation," in this issue.

IMPLEMENTATION

Cognitive aids "off the shelf" (more accurately, off the Internet) are seldom ideal for use in any specific clinical environment. The available resources, operating room physical layout, scope of surgical caseload, and even the important telephone numbers must be addressed in customization of the checklist before introduction into practice. Like the training, this work is best undertaken by a multidisciplinary operating room team whose members each add value from a different perspective. By doing so, the participants develop a sense of ownership of the checklists and become champions for adoption among their own colleagues.

As the world, including the operating room, becomes more and more digital, the choice of paper or digital format for the emergency checklist will arise. This choice is not necessarily an either-or proposition, and providing access to both formats can be an effective strategy. The most critical aspect of this choice relates to how the checklist is accessed for real-time management of critical events. Complementary use of the tools for study, teaching, or case review is probably amenable to multiple formats. The local implementation team will have a good sense of existing workflows in the operating room and whether the operating room team, including but not limited to the anesthesia staff, is accustomed and proficient in the use of digital references during patient care. This reference may take the form of access to the checklist on a smartphone or other personal digital device,[43,44] on a wall-mounted video display panel, or be integrated into an anesthesia information system. In one survey of trainees using the SPA manual in simulation, the users preferred the printed manual to the digital display.[45] Nonetheless, where feasible and acceptable, accessing the cognitive aid on a screen visible to the entire team may have advantages[46] and serve as a physical manifestation of the shared mental model.[47] An assessment of the availability of hardware (monitors, screens, and computers) to be used for this purpose is important and may make evident the possibility that displaying the checklist may take up monitor "real estate" needed for other purposes (eg, physiologic monitoring). At this time, electronic users of these cognitive aids are interacting with static displays of the material. There is considerable interest in the future potential of checklists integrated with sources of data on the patient's condition so that the checklist becomes a dynamic tool.[48] A basic example of this is for the dynamic checklist to provide calculated weight-based drug doses. This promising approach is in its infancy.

The limitations of available hardware are obviously moot when a bound, printed handbook format is adopted. In this case, the key considerations are accessibility, visibility, and awareness of the printed tool's availability and location. Strategies to maintain these handbooks in their proper location are important and include physically securing them in a highly visible place and providing sufficient alternative access to the material so that the need or motivation to pilfer them from the operating room is mitigated.

As noted, the principal purpose of these tools is to support and improve real-time clinical management of critical events. They can be valuable for other purposes, too. Anticipating an event in a patient or procedure where a particular propensity to a complication is recognized, the checklists provide a quick guide to preparing for such an event. Similarly, their use as a teaching tool is a natural adaptation in which their streamlined enumeration of the key, most effective management steps is an excellent foundation for an efficient discussion of uncommon, acute operating room emergencies. After an event, a review of the actual management of the case against the checklist steps can serve as a framework for learning in debriefing, peer review, or morbidity and mortality discussion. In these settings, departments and groups should develop the routine of assessing management of critical events in the framework of the cognitive aid content as part of their case review. The implementation champion, or others, may assume the role of introducing the checklist into the discussion when appropriate. When implementers of the crisis checklists were surveyed, it became evident that a higher frequency of these additional applications increased familiarity and awareness and was associated with a greater reported likelihood of use in acute emergencies: use begets use.[49]

It is clear that achieving reliable use of these tools to improve patient care requires more than printing and distributing the material. The use of these tools demands a cultural change in which humility and collaboration replace autonomy.[1] Achieving this change occurs through a deliberate, multipronged implementation strategy that begins with socializing the use of these aids so that their use becomes standard operating procedure and is not stigmatized or taken as a sign of inadequate expertise. Successful implementers recognize 8 key steps and design a strategy for these that is compatible with their circumstances and capabilities. In addition, the more of these strategies that are undertaken, the more frequently the survey respondents report reliable use[49] (**Box 1**).

The components of an implementation strategy are addressed in detail in the on-line Emergency Manuals Implementation Guide[50] (**Fig. 1**), in which they are each discussed and a variety of resources to support their execution are linked. A valuable early step in the introduction of emergency manuals is for the project team to review each of these implementation steps and determine whether and how each could be used in its particular setting.

SUSTAINING USE

The adoption of crisis checklists in clinical practice is not a once-and-done proposition. The checklists themselves are modified and updated by their authors over

---

Box 1
Cognitive aid implementation steps

- Create buy-in
- Build a multidisciplinary team
- Modify and customize the tools
- Pilot test
- Train staff
- Expand use
- Ongoing training
- Monitor use

---

time, often in response to revisions of the underlying practice guidelines or new evidence informing the management of the specific events. Users are obliged to monitor the sources of their checklists for such updates. Most Web-based checklist download sites request email contact information from the downloader, in part to facilitate outreach when modifications are adopted. At the local level, experience of those using the checklists in clinical care or simulation reveals content that can be improved, and a process for editing the local version of the tools must be established. Some events drive immediate changes to the checklist content, such as a newly recognized contraindication to a treatment or the unavailability of a drug or device referenced in the treatment guidance. The burden and speed of publishing these revisions is substantially lower with electronic tools than with printed manuals. Other changes can be

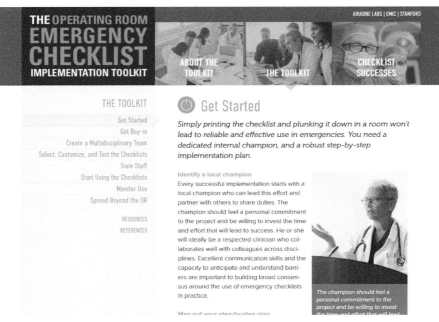

Fig. 1. Emergency manuals implementation guide.

accumulated and incorporated in a regularly scheduled review and revision cycle. These changes include minor changes in formatting or language to improve the clarity and usability of the documents, often based on user feedback. Often, there are clinical situations not addressed in the originally implemented checklist compendium for which there is a need identified in a specific setting. For example, in the author's institution, obstetrics and spine surgery are major clinical areas that the Ariadne checklist compendium did not address, leading us to convene our clinical teams to create these additions to the crisis checklists. Finding an existing checklist for the purpose and adapting it as an addendum may be an option (see **Table 1**). Otherwise, drafting a new checklist for the compendium could be necessary. In this case, key considerations are a multidisciplinary review of relevant existing practice guidelines, extracting the most critical management considerations, and converting these to language appropriate for the checklist while adhering to the layout and design guidance underlying the existing checklists so that those qualities are preserved and a consistent look and "feel" is maintained to promote ease of use. The Implementation Toolkit provides a template for the creation of a new checklist capturing the major design features of the Ariadne Labs crisis checklists.

SUMMARY

Cognitive aids can serve as an antidote to the combined effects of the stress and inevitable unfamiliarity associated with management of rare, high-acuity critical events. As clinicians increasingly appreciate the importance of rescue from such events as a discriminator of the quality of care,[51] both early recognition (see Thomas T. Klumpner and colleagues' article, "Opportunities to Improve Our Capacity to Rescue: Intraoperative and Perioperative Tools," in this issue) and appropriate response are critical components of improving results.[52] These approaches, along with practicing clinicians' preparation with simulated drills and supporting interventions with cognitive aids, represent a modern, multifaceted approach to the care of patients experiencing serious deterioration under medical care.

REFERENCES

1. Gawande A. The checklist manifesto. New York: Henry Holt and Company; 2009.
2. 1993 FDA Anesthesia Machine Pre-Use Check. Available at: https://vam.anest.ufl.edu/fdacheckout.html. Accessed March 12, 2020.
3. Pinyavat T, Wong C, Rosenberg H. Development and evolution of the MHAUS cognitive aid for malignant hyperthermia. BMC Anesthesiol 2014;14(Suppl 1):A25.
4. Babcock WW. Resuscitation during anesthesia. Anesth Analg 1924;3(6):208–13.
5. Haynes AB, Weiser TG, Berry WR, et al. A surgical safety checklist to reduce morbidity and mortality in a global population. N Engl J Med 2009;360(5):491–9.
6. Pronovost P, Needham D, Berenholtz S, et al. An intervention to decrease catheter-related bloodstream infections in the ICU. N Engl J Med 2006;355(26): 2725–32.
7. Delisle M, Pradarelli JC, Panda N, et al. Variation in global uptake of the Surgical Safety Checklist. Br J Surg 2020;107(2):e151–60.
8. Weiser TG, Haynes AB, Lashoher A, et al. Perspectives in quality: designing the WHO Surgical Safety Checklist. Int J Qual Health Care 2010;22(5):365–70.
9. Checklist for Checklists. Available at: https://www.projectcheck.org/uploads/1/0/9/0/1090835/checklist_for_checklists_final_10.3.pdf. Accessed March 30, 2020.

10. Marshall SD, Sanderson P, McIntosh CA, et al. The effect of two cognitive aid designs on team functioning during intra-operative anaphylaxis emergencies: a multi-centre simulation study. Anaesthesia 2016;71(4):389–404.
11. Stanford Anesthesia Cognitive Aid Group. Emergency Manual. Available at: https://emergencymanual.stanford.edu/. Accessed March 30, 2020.
12. Ariadne Labs. OR Crisis Checklists. Available at: https://www.ariadnelabs.org/resources/downloads/. Accessed March 30, 2020.
13. Society for Pediatric Anesthesia. Pedi Crisis 2.0 Critical Events Checklists. Pedi Crisis 2.0 Critical Events Checklists. Available at: https://www.pedsanesthesia.org/critical-events-checklist/. Accessed March 30, 2020.
14. Emergency Manuals Implementation Collaborative: Tools & Resources. Available at: https://www.emergencymanuals.org/tools-resources/. Accessed March 30, 2020.
15. Hoefnagel AL, Rajan S, Martin A, et al. Cognitive aids for the diagnosis and treatment of neuroanesthetic emergencies: consensus guidelines on behalf of the society for neuroscience in anesthesiology and critical care (SNACC) education committee. J Neurosurg Anesthesiol 2019;31(1):7–17.
16. Ziewacz JE, Berven SH, Mummaneni VP, et al. The design, development, and implementation of a checklist for intraoperative neuromonitoring changes. Neurosurg Focus 2012;33(5):E11.
17. Vitale MG, Skaggs DL, Pace GI, et al. Best practices in intraoperative neuromonitoring in spine deformity surgery: development of an intraoperative checklist to optimize response. Spine Deform 2014;2(5):333–9.
18. Neal JM, Mulroy MF, Weinberg GL. American Society of Regional Anesthesia and Pain Medicine. American Society of Regional Anesthesia and Pain Medicine checklist for managing local anesthetic systemic toxicity: 2012 version. Reg Anesth Pain Med 2012;37(1):16–8.
19. ASA Committee on Trauma & Emergency Preparedness. ASA Mass Casualty Checklist. Available at: https://www.asahq.org/-/media/sites/asahq/files/secure/resources/asa-committee-work-products-members-only/or-mass-casualty-checklist.pdf?la=en&hash=FA1B5AF93861D423EF0548C327BE4C65F746AB1D. Accessed March 13, 2020.
20. Nepple KG, Sandhu GS, Rogers CG, et al. Description of a multicenter safety checklist for intraoperative hemorrhage control while clamped during robotic partial nephrectomy. Patient Saf Surg 2012;6:8.
21. Katheria A, Rich W, Finer N. Development of a strategic process using checklists to facilitate team preparation and improve communication during neonatal resuscitation. Resuscitation 2013;84(11):1552–7.
22. Tobin JM, Grabinsky A, McCunn M, et al. A checklist for trauma and emergency anesthesia. Anesth Analg 2013;117(5):1178–84.
23. Malignant Hyperthermia Association of the United States (MHAUS). Emergency Therapy for MH. 2019. Available at: https://my.mhaus.org/store/ViewProduct.aspx?id=1512933. Accessed March 12, 2020.
24. Tarola CL, Hirji S, Yule SJ, et al. Cognitive support to promote shared mental models during safety-critical situations in cardiac surgery (late breaking report). IEEE Conf Cogn Comput Asp Situat Manag Cogsima (2018) 2018;2018:165–7.
25. Quick Reference Handbook. Association of Anaesthetists of Great Britain & Ireland. Available at: https://anaesthetists.org/Home/Resources-publications/Safety-alerts/Anaesthesia-emergencies/Quick-Reference-Handbook. Accessed March 13, 2020.

26. Stanford Cognitive Aids in Medicine. OB Anesthesia Emergency Manual. Available at: http://med.stanford.edu/cogaids/obanesem.html. Accessed March 13, 2020.
27. Borshoff D. The anaesthetic crisis manual; 2011.
28. Gaba DM, Fish KJ, Howard SK, et al. Crisis management in anesthesiology E-book. Elsevier Health Sciences; 2014.
29. Chu LF, Fuller A. A visual guide to crisis management. Philadelphia: Lippincott Williams & Wilkins; 2012.
30. Morell RC, Cooper JB. APSF sponsors workshop on implementing emergency manuals. Philadelphia: Anesthesia Patient Safety Foundation Newsletter; 2016. Available at: https://www.apsf.org/article/apsf-sponsors-workshop-on-implementing-emergency-manuals/. Accessed March 13, 2020.
31. Arriaga AF, Bader AM, Wong JM, et al. Simulation-based trial of surgical-crisis checklists. N Engl J Med 2013;368(3):246–53.
32. Neal JM, Hsiung RL, Mulroy MF, et al. ASRA checklist improves trainee performance during a simulated episode of local anesthetic systemic toxicity. Reg Anesth Pain Med 2012;37(1):8–15.
33. Harrison TK, Manser T, Howard SK, et al. Use of cognitive aids in a simulated anesthetic crisis. Anesth Analg 2006;103(3):551–6.
34. Hardy J-B, Gouin A, Damm C, et al. The use of a checklist improves anaesthesiologists' technical and non-technical performance for simulated malignant hyperthermia management. Anaesth Crit Care Pain Med 2018;37(1):17–23.
35. Burden AR, Carr ZJ, Staman GW, et al. Does every code need a "reader?" improvement of rare event management with a cognitive aid "reader" during a simulated emergency: a pilot study. Simul Healthc 2012;7(1):1–9.
36. Greenberg CC, Regenbogen SE, Studdert DM, et al. Patterns of communication breakdowns resulting in injury to surgical patients. J Am Coll Surg 2007;204(4):533–40.
37. Mazzocco K, Petitti DB, Fong KT, et al. Surgical team behaviors and patient outcomes. Am J Surg 2009;197(5):678–85.
38. Mills PD, DeRosier JM, Neily J, et al. A cognitive aid for cardiac arrest: you can't use it if you don't know about it. Jt Comm J Qual Saf 2004;30(9):488–96.
39. Kolb DA. Experience as the source of learning and development. Upper Saddle River (NJ): Prentice Hall; 1984.
40. Goldhaber-Fiebert SN, Lei V, Nandagopal K, et al. Emergency manual implementation: can brief simulation-based or staff trainings increase familiarity and planned clinical use? Jt Comm J Qual Patient Saf 2015;41(5):212–20.
41. Guise J-M, Mladenovic J. In situ simulation: identification of systems issues. Semin Perinatol 2013;37(3):161–5.
42. Delisle M, Pradarelli JC, Panda N, et al. Methods for scaling simulation-based teamwork training. BMJ Qual Saf 2020;29(2):98–102.
43. Schild S, Sedlmayr B, Schumacher A-K, et al. A digital cognitive aid for anesthesia to support intraoperative crisis management: results of the user-centered design process. JMIR Mhealth Uhealth 2019;7(4):e13226.
44. McEvoy MD, Hand WR, Stoll WD, et al. Adherence to guidelines for the management of local anesthetic systemic toxicity is improved by an electronic decision support tool and designated "Reader". Reg Anesth Pain Med 2014;39(4):299–305.
45. Watkins SC, Anders S, Clebone A, et al. Paper or plastic? Simulation based evaluation of two versions of a cognitive aid for managing pediatric peri-operative

critical events by anesthesia trainees: evaluation of the society for pediatric anesthesia emergency checklist. J Clin Monit Comput 2016;30(3):275–83.

46. Mainthia R, Lockney T, Zotov A, et al. Novel use of electronic whiteboard in the operating room increases surgical team compliance with pre-incision safety practices. Surgery 2012;151(5):660–6.

47. Wu L, Cirimele J, Card S, et al. Maintaining shared mental models in anesthesia crisis care with nurse tablet input and large-screen displays. In Proceedings of the 24th annual ACM symposium adjunct on User interface software and technology (UIST '11 Adjunct). New York: Association for Computing Machinery; 2011. p. 71–2. https://doi.org/10.1145/2046396.2046428.

48. Robbins J, Schaffer GN, Cohen BJ, et al. Patent Pending US20140006943A1 - Operating room checklist system - Google Patents. 2014.

49. Alidina S, Goldhaber-Fiebert SN, Hannenberg AA, et al. Factors associated with the use of cognitive aids in operating room crises: a cross-sectional study of US hospitals and ambulatory surgical centers. Implement Sci 2018;13(1):50.

50. Emergency Manuals Implementation Guide. Available at: http://implementingemergencymanuals.org. Accessed March 7, 2020.

51. Ghaferi AA, Birkmeyer JD, Dimick JB. Complications, failure to rescue, and mortality with major inpatient surgery in medicare patients. Ann Surg 2009;250(6): 1029–34.

52. Taenzer AH, Pyke JB, McGrath SP. A review of current and emerging approaches to address failure-to-rescue. Anesthesiology 2011;115(2):421–31.

Real-Time Debriefing After Critical Events

Exploring the Gap Between Principle and Reality

Alexander F. Arriaga, MD, MPH, ScD[a,b,c],*, Demian Szyld, MD, EdM[d,e],
May C.M. Pian-Smith, MD, MS[e,f]

KEYWORDS

- Critical event debriefing • Debriefing • Feedback • Patient safety
- Medical education • Crew/crisis resource management • Medical simulation
- Implementation science

KEY POINTS

- Debriefing after perioperative critical events potentially benefits the individual, team, environment, and overall health care system.
- In studies of actual critical events across medical disciplines, debriefing only takes place a fraction of the time.
- The implementation sciences, as well as recent implementation research pertaining to patient safety interventions, may provide insight toward closing the gap between principle and reality.

INTRODUCTION

Perioperative crises (eg, cardiac arrest, massive hemorrhage) are life-threatening events that can have a secondary impact on the providers themselves.[1] Our understanding of the incidence of these crises is limited by variations in reporting requirements, definitions, and other factors. Based on safety reporting, available data suggest an incidence of 145 in 10,000 cases.[2] With the global volume of surgery estimated at 313 million procedures per year,[3,4] the burden of associated crises may be in the millions annually.[5] Yet, these events can be rare at the level of individual providers,

[a] Department of Anesthesiology, Perioperative and Pain Medicine, Brigham and Women's Hospital, 75 Francis Street, Boston, MA 02115, USA; [b] Ariadne Labs, Boston, MA, USA; [c] Center for Surgery and Public Health, Boston, MA, USA; [d] Department of Emergency Medicine, Brigham and Women's Hospital, 75 Francis Street, Boston, MA 02115, USA; [e] Center for Medical Simulation, Boston, MA, USA; [f] Department of Anesthesia, Critical Care & Pain Medicine, Massachusetts General Hospital, 55 Fruit Street, Boston, MA 02114, USA
* Corresponding author. Department of Anesthesiology, Perioperative and Pain Medicine, Brigham and Women's Hospital, 75 Francis Street, Boston, MA 02115.
E-mail address: aarriaga@post.harvard.edu
Twitter: @alexarriaga1234 (A.F.A.); @debriefmentor (D.S.)

Anesthesiology Clin 38 (2020) 801–820
https://doi.org/10.1016/j.anclin.2020.08.003
1932-2275/20/© 2020 Elsevier Inc. All rights reserved.
anesthesiology.theclinics.com

which only adds to their potential to induce stress, be complex to manage, and affect provider burnout and wellness. In a national survey of the impact of perioperative catastrophes on anesthesiologists, 84% of respondents noted they had been involved in at least 1 unanticipated death or serious injury over the course of their career, with 19% acknowledging they had never fully recovered.[1] Further, these estimates of incidence do not include disruptive clinician behavior that undermines a culture of safety,[6] critical communication breakdowns,[7] events that become critical in the setting of a pandemic,[8] and other critical events that have gained increased attention for their impact on providers.

Debriefing after critical events is supported by decades of literature in medicine and other high-stakes industries.[9–16] Yet, in studies of actual clinical practice and critical events, a gap exists between principle and reality. In studies across medical disciplines, debriefing after critical events only takes place a fraction of the time.[7,17,18]

The purpose of this article is to explore this gap and facilitate the ability of readers to address the chasm. This article focuses on debriefing shortly after a critical event or the associated operation/procedure (ie, proximal debriefing; "hot" debriefing).[19] For more on debriefing nomenclature in the context of the scope of this article, see **Box 1**. We seek to explore the growing suspicion[7,17,18] that "nothing debriefing" (ie, no debriefing) is taking place after countless perioperative crises internationally, and search for ways to improve this gap where indicated. This discussion will hopefully allow the reader to take a self-directed and locally customized approach toward best practices.

PART I: THE POTENTIAL BENEFITS FROM DEBRIEFING

Potential benefits of debriefing can affect individuals, cross-disciplinary groups and teams, and an entire system. Debriefing can both provide 360° feedback to team members and address all of the residency core competencies from Accreditation Council for Graduate Medical Education, including medical knowledge, patient care, practice-based learning, interpersonal skills and communication, professionalism, and systems-based practice.[13] Debriefing can facilitate mastery learning for events such as advanced cardiac life support and pediatric advanced life support.[42] It plays a central role in experiential learning environments, such as medical simulation, with debriefing frameworks that have been designed and adapted for clinical environments.[30,43–46] It has also been used as a vehicle to identify systems gaps and improve patient safety and quality.[16] There are at least 2 reasons why debriefing critical events may have important benefits to the health care system. First, by listening to frontline clinicians, administrators and leaders can learn about the difference between "work as imagined" and "work as done."[47] Workarounds are very common in health care and can undermine safety processes.[48] Second, organizational learning from celebrating successes is critical to sustaining resilience. Whereas errors and near misses can be reported to highlight safety threats, practices that contribute to safety are not frequently reported. These events can be deliberately solicited when teams debrief critical events and resuscitations. Leaders of health systems that implemented successful debriefing programs reported that "the debrief aims to identify and address flaws in the system and improve patient safety and system function." Debriefing leads to "addressing concerns that impacted the teams' ability to perform its job efficiently in addition to other issues related to improving performance. The fact that issues of equipment and process could be corrected, and the surgical team could experience the immediate benefits of participation, gave them a greater commitment to the process."[49]

Box 1
Debriefing nomenclature in the context of the scope of this article

The scope of this article is targeted at debriefing after critical events and the elusive gap that exists between principle and reality. This article is not meant to be a "how-to" for critical event debriefing or a review of different debriefing methods; there are existing texts that cover this.[20,21] It is also not meant as a dedicated article on the implementation sciences,[22–27] although some of this will be covered for its invaluable place in the conversation. In terms of nomenclature, we will draw some of our definitions from the American Heart Association Scientific Statement made by Cheng and colleagues:

> Most literature blurs the line between feedback and debriefing.[28] Although this line remains indistinct, available definitions differentiate them. Here, we view data as a form of objective unprocessed information that makes up feedback. Thus, feedback is defined as information about the performance compared with a standard[29] (eg, automatically generated data from simulators or devices that capture the quality of CPR). Debriefing is a reflective conversation about performance and may include processed select performance data (ie, feedback).[30,31] Finally, performance refers to both taskwork and teamwork.[32] Taskwork represents what the team does, such as adhering to a resuscitation algorithm, but also includes psychomotor skills, such as performing CPR or defibrillation; teamwork reflects how team members perform taskwork with each other.[32]

This article is focused on proximal, or "hot" debriefing, that is, debriefing at the point of care shortly after a critical event or the associated operation/procedure.[19] This article is not specifically focused on routine debriefing after every single case,[33,34] although this broader strategy would invariably include cases where there was a critical event. Indeed, there is evidence that interventions that involve routine debriefing after every case can improve patient and other outcomes if successfully implemented.[35–38] Salient research and implementation lessons from routine debriefing is discussed where appropriate, while attempting to keep critical event debriefing at the center of this review.

This article is not exclusive to critical incident stress debriefing, which is mentioned as a type of debriefing after critical events and has a valuable role in the topic of debriefing overall.[12,39,40] An entire article can be written exploring the foundations and theories of different debriefing approaches, and there is growing literature on the considerable commonality that now exists between feedback and debriefing, with a call for future work regarding the relevance of integrating these concepts where appropriate.[41]

Data from Refs.[12,19–41]

Another key benefit of debriefing is its ability to identify and potentially mitigate the negative impact that critical events can have on health care providers. In a national survey of anesthesiologists regarding perioperative catastrophic events, more than 70% of those reporting a "most memorable" perioperative catastrophe experienced guilt, anxiety, and reliving of the event; 88% required time to recover emotionally and 19% noted they never fully recovered. Overall, 89% of respondents felt that debriefing with the entire operating room (OR) team would be helpful to providers in the future, and 68% felt the resource should be a standard operating procedure.[1] In a separate survey study of consultant anesthesiologists in Australia, who were presented with a hypothetical crisis scenario, the majority agreed or strongly agreed that there should be a formal strategy for anesthesiologists to deal with the aftermath, and 83% agreed or strongly agreed that "debriefing the OR team immediately after a perioperative death is advisable."[12] Similar results were found in a survey study of anesthesiologists in Canada regarding their experience with unanticipated perioperative deaths.[50]

These findings are particularly important in this era of attention to provider well-being and burnout.[51–53] Clinicians are already at the forefront of absorbing the hazards of crisis events, sometimes with the label of "hero," as they protect patients from an imperfect system.[54,55] During the coronavirus disease-19 (COVID-19) pandemic, there were 18 anesthesiologists and 2 anesthesia nurses in China who became known as the "coronavirus intubation team racing against death," who performed nearly 50 intubations over 8 days for patients with severe COVID-19.[8] In the setting of this and other events, the Chinese Society of Anesthesiology and the Chinese Association of Anesthesiologists jointly established a platform for free mental health advice to all anesthesia providers[8]; one can envision the role debriefing can play in this process. Despite all the potential benefits from debriefing, it is acknowledged that health care providers should not be forced to debrief, because some people may recover best with solitude and isolation,[12] and more involved forms of debriefing (such as critical incident stress debriefing)[39,40] could have unintended iatrogenic effects.[56] Overall, the reported potential benefits of debriefing after critical events have been largely positive across an international sample of providers.

PART II: THE LANDSCAPE AND SCARCITY OF THIS PRACTICE AFTER ACTUAL CRITICAL EVENTS

Despite the long history of debriefing in medicine and other high-stakes industries, there is growing evidence that the rate of debriefing after perioperative crises is far from 100%. Our understanding is hindered in part owing to the paucity of research studying actual critical events (vs simulated or hypothetical events). This likely stems from the unpredictable, often sudden, and relatively infrequent occurrence of perioperative crises compared with overall surgical and procedural volumes. Nevertheless, even survey research can yield great insight. In the survey study of Canadian anesthesiologists registered with the College of Physicians and Surgeons of Alberta (ie, not specific to trainees) regarding unanticipated perioperative deaths, only 14% of those reporting an unanticipated perioperative death participated in an OR debriefing or other immediate process.[50] No specific reason for this lack of debriefing was provided, although themes from free-text participant comments called for formal policies for support of OR team members and encouragement for support that was individualized to specific needs.

This phenomenon is not specific to anesthesiology or even the perioperative space. A brief summary of selected literature can be found in **Box 2**. There is a common finding that "hot" debriefs in clinical settings are infrequent, and the barriers noted in studies and other publications (including "too many urgent patient care issues," lack of trained debriefing facilitators [which may influence willingness to facilitate/debrief], fear of judgment from colleagues, discomfort regarding the event, lack of administrative support, and overall buy-in)[13,18,57,58] may resonate with members of a perioperative team who struggle with constraints of production pressure, coupled with limited time and space, in busy surgical and procedural areas.

In addition to these survey studies, our understanding is enhanced by mixed-methods research that includes semistructured interviews of participants shortly after actual critical events. In a study of critical events experienced by anesthesiology residents at a large academic medical center over a 1-year period,[7] only 49% of the events were associated with at least some bare minimum components of a proximal debriefing that included the study participant. Only 39% of events occurred in the OR (ie, main OR locations excluding obstetric ORs and non-OR anesthesia locations), which speaks to both the rapid expansion of non-OR anesthesia, as well as the

---

Box 2
Lessons from selected medical literature not specific to anesthesiology on the landscape and scarcity of debriefing after actual critical events

- A national survey of pediatric emergency medicine fellows regarding critically ill children in the emergency department (ED) showed that 99% of respondents had participated in medical resuscitations during their fellowship, yet more than 30% indicated that they had never participated in a debriefing session afterward; the majority estimated that postresuscitation debriefing in the ED took place 50% or less of the time. Although the reasons for this were unclear, 88% of respondents reported no formal teaching on how to debrief, and 87% noted that their fellowship program did not have a structured format for debriefing.[18]

- A survey of staff from Canadian pediatric EDs (nurses, fellows, and attending physicians) revealed that 52.5% of respondents indicated that debriefing after real resuscitations occurred less than 25% of the time, and 63% had no previous training in debriefing. More than 90% of respondents indicated workload and time shortages as debriefing barriers.[58]

- In a study on the implementation of a debriefing tool for emergent resuscitations in a pediatric ED, there was a 26% debriefing rate after the critical events of interest (cardiopulmonary resuscitation, intubation, and/or defibrillation), and "too many urgent patient care issues" was identified as a theme in cases not debriefed.[57]

- In a survey of resuscitation training officers (physicians [house officers (including in anesthesia) and registrars], nurses, and other team members responding to in-hospital cardiac arrest) across the United Kingdom, less than 8% of respondents said they completed a formal debrief after a cardiac arrest. The reasons for this were again unclear, although the majority of respondents noted that debrief sessions were either offered but not taken up, or were very informal, often limited to a few members of team.[59]

- In a survey study of Canadian internal medicine residents, only 5.9% of cardiac arrest teams reported receiving postevent debriefing and only 1.3% reported getting performance feedback. Although the respondents did not report a reason, more than 85% reported that postcardiac arrest debriefing would indeed be effective or very effective for improving their skills and confidence.[17]

Data from Refs.[17,18,57–59]

---

ubiquitous presence of anesthesia providers throughout the health system. For any scalable intervention to improve critical event debriefing for an entire team, the anesthesia provider could be in a unique position to spread the intervention across the OR, non-OR anesthesia locations, intensive care units, labor and delivery, code teams, trauma alert teams, and other areas. The authors also studied critical events that involved disruptive behavior and critical communication breakdowns; they found that the presence of a critical communication breakdown was significantly associated with the event not being debriefed (illustrative vignettes of these breakdowns are shown in **Table 1**). This finding supports the notion that barriers to debriefing are not just related to time, space, resources, training, production pressure, or even belief in the value of debriefing overall. There may be social and interpersonal factors at play regarding whether proximal debriefing is viable, or at the very least whether it is likely to happen easily.

This mixed-methods study was followed up with a qualitative study that further explored the interviews with anesthesia residents after actual critical events.[60] The interviews revealed that debriefing for the residents, in the setting of real events, was considered part of a multistage process that included internal dialogue, event documentation (as a component of reconstructing what happened), and lessons they felt they learned (not necessarily in this order or with distinct borders). In each stage of

Table 1
Critical communication breakdowns observed and illustrative vignettes from mixed-methods study of debriefing after real critical events[7]

Category	Description	Illustrative Vignette
Audience failure	Key person missing from a critical Conversation	"Profound desaturation after resident extubated patient at the end of a case. A second on-call anesthesia resident incidentally was also present for extubation … neither of us had a free hand. And I think at some point, I don't remember exactly when it was, we asked the circulator, can you please call our attending. And she couldn't reach our attending. She called the wrong attending."
Occasion failure	A key discussion that became futile to poor timing or a lack of communication of a key piece of clinical information during the event	A critically ill patient scheduled for an elective case transported directly to the OR without communication between relevant parties involved. No tracing on the arterial line (unclear timing of this); massive pulmonary embolism suspected.
Content failure	Insufficient or inaccurate information regarding critical details	Elective case canceled in preoperative holding area after 3 hours of attempted coordination and data gathering involving an adult patient with congenital heart disease
Purpose failure	Failure to resolve a critical issue that was discussed, or discontent/disagreement with another clinician regarding a critical issue	Strong disagreement between nurse and anesthesia resident regarding the administration of naloxone during a request for intubation of a patient in the hospital ward. Two additional requests for intubation of patients in the hospital occurred right after this incident. Never was addressed.
Systems failure	Lapse in communication at the organizational level	Obstetric emergency ("level 1") called on the labor and delivery floor; pagers were down. This led to a delay in the discussion between the anesthesia and obstetric teams regarding critical information.

From Arriaga AF, Sweeney RE, Clapp JT, et al. Failure to Debrief after Critical Events in Anesthesia Is Associated with Failures in Communication during the Event. Anesthesiology 2019;130(6):1039-1048; Table 2, p.1043; with permission.

this process, there were residents who were self-negotiating their perceived reputation, affective response, and extent to which they internally felt culpable for what had happened. One resident being interviewed after a critical event pondered "if things would have gone differently" if they themselves had been better prepared. Another resident intentionally avoided discussing the critical event out of fear that colleagues may judge them: "Why is this incompetent resident asking so many questions right now? ...especially since I was in the mindset of blaming myself for the situation." In the medical literature, debriefing is noted for its ability to mitigate shame and blame and embrace patient safety and the medical simulation principle of respecting a predefined basic assumption regarding the ability and engagement of participants (a popular basic assumption in simulation and debriefing is that, "We believe that everyone participating in this simulation is intelligent, capable, cares about doing their best, and wants to improve").[21,27,61] Despite an abundance of medical literature supporting the ability of debriefing to directly address these resident concerns of reputation, culpability, and affective response, the rate of debriefing after critical events in this study was only 49%, which (based on the literature) may even overestimate how frequently debriefing is taking place more broadly. This finding supports the cultural barriers that have been noted by others less directly via needs assessment surveys and editorials.[13,58] These issues go well beyond getting leadership to buy-in; obtaining time, space, and resources; and addressing production pressure. To truly close this gap, there will likely need to be more research that involves lessons from both medical simulation and actual events at the point of care. Some of this may involve getting a better understanding of what providers are actually learning and/or changing, at the point of care, as the result of a proximal debriefing. In the words of the teamwork and patient safety experts Salas and colleagues,[27] "Even if this [debriefing, especially after critical events] lasts for as little as 3 minutes, it is important to be able to discuss the relevant event(s) and the observed teamwork behaviors in an environment that is, safe from administrative oversight where the focus must be on gaining information, understanding, and insight." Perhaps the synthesis of the gap between the medical literature and reality is best summarized by an editorial by Pian-Smith and Cooper (**Box 3**).

PART III: THE BRIDGE BETWEEN PRINCIPLE AND REALITY: STRATEGIES TO OFFER OPPORTUNITIES FOR REFLECTION ON ACTUAL CRITICAL EVENTS
The Implementation Sciences

The implementation sciences represent an important field of study to leverage when introducing real-time debriefing into actual clinical practice. As nomenclature, we provide some terminology offered by Rapport and colleagues (**Box 4**).

Rapport has placed several of these concepts into a schematic, showing an interconnected feedback loop that can be created across 5 surrounding categories (**Fig. 1**). There is a large range of literature available relevant to local implementation of a patient safety intervention, including introductory overviews of the field[66]; systematic and literature reviews[25,67]; studies that work toward common definitions, frameworks, and categories[68,69]; and step-by-step implementation checklists and processes.[70,71] There are also works specific to patient safety interventions and/or

---

Box 3
Excerpt from 2019 Editorial by Pian-Smith and Cooper regarding debriefing after real critical events[62]

We strongly believe that routine debriefing after all critical events is the right thing to do. However, we acknowledge that there is not good evidence or experience for how best to do it. There is evidence that our debriefings, as they stand now, are not ideal: participants can be left feeling more personally responsible, blamed, depressed, and fearful.[1] We have much to learn about how to make the debriefs safe, effective, and practical....These and other questions can best be answered with research on this topic, perhaps much of it in the natural environment during real debriefings and also via simulation.

Data from Refs.[1,62]

Box 4
Nomenclature from the implementation sciences (from Rapport and colleagues)[26]

Implementation science, dissemination and implementation (D&I),[63] evidence-based interventional dissemination,[64] and implementation research,[65] is a basket of terms that refers to the application of effective and evidence-based interventions, in targeted settings, to improve the health and well-being of specific population groups. Implementation science is the scientific study of methods that take findings into practice, while 'effective implementation' refers to the process whereby an actionable plan is appropriately and successfully executed.

Data from Refs.[26,63–65]

---

debriefing, not all of which are exclusive to the implementation sciences, where lessons salient to implementing critical event debriefing can be gathered.[22–24,27,72] This literature, some of which is reviewed elsewhere in this article, should be considered a foundation toward the development of an implementation plan.

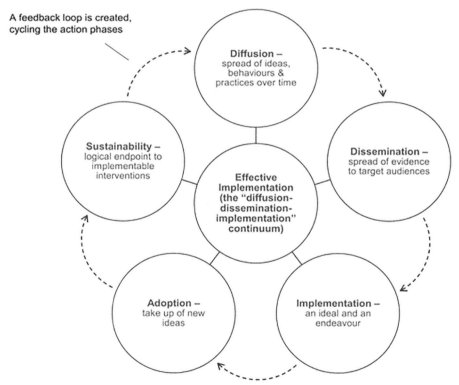

Fig. 1. Five foundational categories of implementation science.[26] (*From* Rapport F, Clay-Williams R, Churruca K, et al. The struggle of translating science into action: Foundational concepts of implementation science. J Eval Clin Pract 2018;24(1):117-126. Figure 1, p. 119. With permission.)

The literature on implementation sciences (some of which is not necessarily specific to medicine) offers tremendous insight toward the development of a roadmap to implement change in the field of critical event debriefing. In 2012, Meyers and colleagues[70] described the critical steps of implementation as part of a quality improvement framework comprising 14 interrelated steps across 4 phases (**Fig. 2**). One can imagine putting the contents of **Fig. 2** on a large dry-erase board as a template to map out a strategy specific to a debriefing program customized to one's own institution. It is hard to argue against the value of conducting a needs assessment, determining available resources, and getting buy-in from key stakeholders. Several of these strategies have also been associated with successful implementation of other patient safety interventions, including tools for debriefing.[23,24,57] The essential role of hospital leaders and resources was emphasized in a review by Salas and colleagues[27] on a set of evidence-based best practices and tips for debriefing medical teams.

In a systematic review of targeted literature at the intersection of implementation science and quality/patient safety, Braithwaite and colleagues[25] derived 8 success factors of implementation (**Box 5**). Although the factors in **Box 5** are more overarching and may require more heavy lifting than the schematic approach in **Fig. 2**, they may offer greater potential for longer term planning, rapid cycle improvements, and sustainability. The Consolidated Framework for Implementation Research, the Expert Recommendation for Implementing Change, and Gagliardi and colleagues[71] publications have offered implementation strategy typologies, terms, checklists and/or definitions for those seeking a much more comprehensive list to consider for applicability (such as whether one is at the stage of broad and/or global implementation, such as mass media campaigns and creating debriefing tools in different languages).[66,68,69]

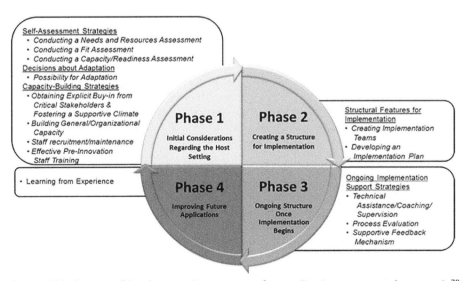

Fig. 2. Critical steps of implementation as part of a quality improvement framework.[70] (*From* Meyers DC, Durlak JA, Wandersman A. The quality implementation framework: a synthesis of critical steps in the implementation process. Am J Community Psychol 2012;50(3-4):462-480. Figure 2, p. 475; with permission.)

Box 5
Success factors for implementation to improve care quality and patient safety (Braithwaite and colleagues[25])

1. Preparing for change (planning from the organization and associated staff).

2. Assessing capacity for implementation, both in terms of people (ie, presence of individuals skilled in the initiative being implemented) and setting (see factor 3).

3. Setting (ie, a setting that is capable of and receptive to change).

4. Choosing the right type of implementation (examples include guidelines, reminders, alerts, checklists, and/or cultural changes).

5. Obtaining resources needed for implementation.

6. Leverage (ie, harnessing key individuals, such as opinion leaders, champions, and change agents).

7. Desirable implementation enabling features (a mosaic of factors including communication, incentives, feedback, and customization to organization/staff needs).

8. Sustainability (including a commitment for ongoing support at a managerial level).

Data from Braithwaite J, Marks D, Taylor N. Harnessing implementation science to improve care quality and patient safety: a systematic review of targeted literature. Int J Qual Health Care 2014;26(3):321-329.

LESSONS FROM THE IMPLEMENTATION OF CRISIS CHECKLISTS AND EMERGENCY MANUALS

There are patient safety tools with associated implementation research, namely, crisis checklists and emergency manuals, that have a natural and logical connection to critical event debriefing given their role to aid in the management of critical events. Crisis checklists, emergency manuals, and other cognitive aids for anesthesia crisis management have existed for decades,[73–77] and they have an even broader reach in their use in aviation and other high-stakes industries.[78] The emergency manual produced by the Stanford Anesthesia Cognitive Aid Group has 2 dedicated pages devoted to key points in crisis resource management,[79] and the book by Gaba and colleagues[73] on crisis management in anesthesiology (which catalogs the management of 99 critical events in anesthesiology) has a dedicated article on debriefing. Goldhaber-Fiebert and Howard[80] popularized 4 vital elements for widespread development and implementation of emergency manuals (which may be valuable in extending these resources to formal debriefing tools): create, familiarize, use, and integrate. In 2013, a simulation-based randomized controlled trial of surgical crisis checklists was published in the *New England Journal of Medicine* reporting that use of crisis checklists was associated with nearly a 75% reduction in failure to adhere to critical steps in management.[81] The Emergency Manuals Implementation Collaborative has subsequently been created to foster the adoption and effective use of emergency manuals to enhance patient safety.[82] We provide a brief paragraph elsewhere in this article on specific suggestions at the intersection of crisis checklists and emergency manuals and critical event debriefing. For more information on cognitive aids in the management of critical events and other salient lessons for implementation, see the publication by Hannenberg,[83] as well as the OR Emergency Checklist Implementation Toolkit.[84]

Building on the thought that perioperative critical events could trigger a debriefing, an institution, department and/or division can identify the specific types of events that should prompt a member of the team to offer a debriefing, or at the very least to screen

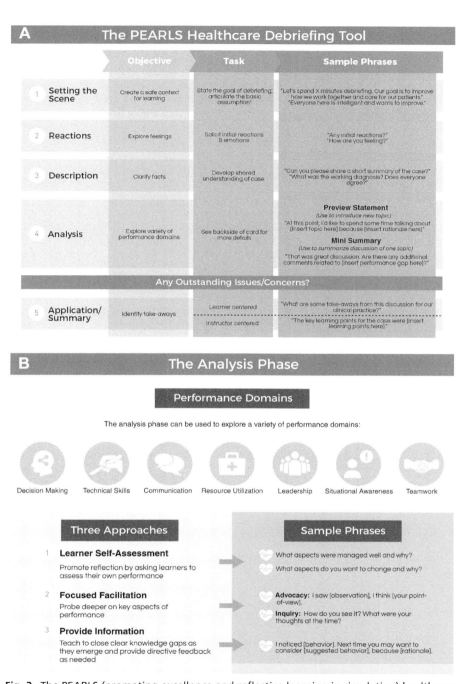

Fig. 3. The PEARLS (promoting excellence and reflective learning in simulation) health care debriefing tool.[44] (*A*): Front; (*B*): Back. (*From* Bajaj K, Meguerdichian M, Thoma B, et al. The PEARLS Healthcare Debriefing Tool. Acad Med 2018;93(2):336. Page 336; with permission.)

for matters that should be addressed before the next case; provide psychological first aid and/or improve awareness of local peer support and employee assistance resources; and assess if team members are able to continue providing care. Similar to how damage control surgery or resuscitation can have a set of goals,[85] "hot" debriefing may provide an opportunity to address certain issues acutely salient to the critical event, the next case, and/or rest of the day or night. The strategy of defining critical events to prompt at least brief communication and debriefing has been described in both the fields of emergency medicine and surgery, with advice to consider starting with events that are most common and/or relevant to staff.[20,86] Based on more recent work studying debriefing after real critical events in anesthesia, one may also want to consider categories for disruptive behavior that undermines a culture of safety,[6] critical communication breakdowns,[86–89] and any event for which an individual specifically requests a debriefing.[7] There is also emerging research to suggest synergy between the implementation of crisis checklists and emergency manuals and critical event debriefing. In a cross-sectional study of US hospitals and ambulatory surgery centers, more successful implementation of crisis checklists and emergency manuals was associated with the use of these tools to aid in debriefing after a critical event.[23] In an institutional case report of implementing emergency manuals, teams were encouraged to debrief using the emergency manuals when events occurred.[24]

Specific Debriefing Tools and Training Programs

We purposefully leave this section brief, because the scope of this article is not to prescribe a specific debriefing method or give a "how-to" for debriefing. It would be the

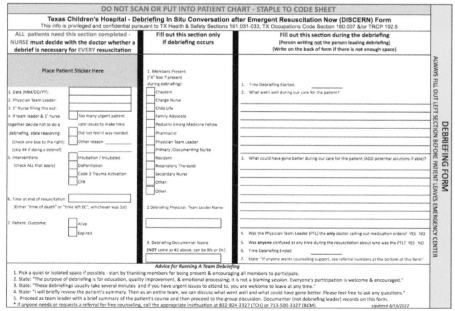

Fig. 4. The DISCERN (debriefing in situ conversation after emergent resuscitation) tool.[57] (*From* Mullan PC, Wuestner E, Kerr TD, et al. Implementation of an in situ qualitative debriefing tool for resuscitations. Resuscitation 2013;84(7):946-951. Figure 1, p. 948; with permission.)

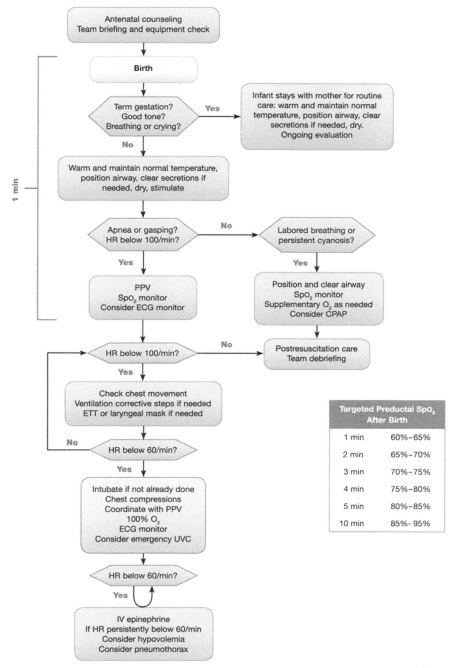

Fig. 5. Neonatal resuscitation algorithm (American Heart Association. 2015 update).[98] (Reprinted with permission from Wyckoff MH, Aziz K, Escobedo MB, et al. Part 13: Neonatal Resuscitation: 2015 American Heart Association Guidelines Update for Cardiopulmonary Resuscitation and Emergency Cardiovascular Care. Circulation 2015;132(18 Suppl 2):S543-560. Figure 1, page S544. © 2015 American Heart Association, Inc.)

subject of an entire article, chapter, and/or series to thoroughly review this. Nevertheless, given the importance of this topic, we provide some literature to allow the reader to customize existing debriefing tools and resources into locally relevant versions. An action card containing items to consider after a real critical event (including debriefing) has been developed based on thousands of incident reports from anesthetists in Australia and New Zealand.[90] Debriefing courses, based on decades of experience and thousands of debriefings of health care simulation, are offered by various programs, for example, the Center for Medical Simulation.[91,92]

Alternatives to traditional high-fidelity simulation have also been explored. Widespread scaling and/or local customization of debriefing programs can invariably involve barriers referred by Delisle and colleagues[93] as the "Three Ts" (training, technology, and time). These barriers may be particularly relevant for areas with limited access to simulation centers and/or specific needs to match local resources. Delisle and Hannenberg review options including telesimulation and teledebriefing, 2 modalities that may become increasingly relevant, even for high-fidelity simulation centers, in the COVID-19 era and beyond. For those seeking more summative information, a review article on different debriefing methods, as well as a conceptual framework for the development of debriefing skills, have been published, and both provide invaluable content to inform educational practice.[21,94]

There are also specific debriefing tools and other resources. The Promoting Excellence And Reflective Learning approach to debriefing has been developed for simulation-based education and adapted in the form of a health care debriefing tool/cognitive aid (**Fig. 3**; this tool has since been translated into multiple languages; as of this publication, the latest version is available at debrief2learn.org).[43,44,95] Specific to point-of-care debriefing after emergent resuscitations, the Debriefing In Situ Conversation after Emergent Resuscitation Now tool has been developed, and its implementation has been tested in an emergency department setting (**Fig. 4**).[57] There are many approaches to debriefing and no comparative studies to suggest that one may be better than another.[21] Kessler and colleagues[20] describe that although physicians are the most common debriefer, social workers and other clinicians can also debrief. Debriefing after clinical events may be led by nurses with minimal prior training.[96] The TALK debrief (https://www.talkdebrief.org), funded by the European Union, is trying to lower barriers by decreasing the need to train facilitators and encouraging all health care personnel to begin a debriefing. We recommend individuals and institutions select 1 approach to debriefing that they find useful and focus on mastery by, for example, developing a peer coaching approach.[97]

SUMMARY

Debriefing after perioperative critical events potentially benefits the individual, team, environment, and overall health care system. At the point of care, there is still a noticeable gap to making this ritual a reliable occurrence. Future work will need to be done, both via medical simulation and actual critical events, to learn how to make point-of-care debriefing safe, effective, and practical,[62] and how to achieve broad implementation, improvement and sustainability. Debriefing deserves the same level of importance as other aspects of managing a critical event. In the American Heart Association Guidelines for Neonatal Resuscitation, "team debriefing" is a key step highlighted in their popular cognitive aid (**Fig. 5**).[98] The American Heart Association scientific statement on resuscitation education science places prominent emphasis on feedback and debriefing.[15] As the popularity grows for resuscitation algorithms specific to anesthesiologists and perioperative teams,[76] perioperative providers and procedure teams can have broad influence on reshaping how the aftermath of critical events are handled at the point of care.

ACKNOWLEDGMENTS

Supported by a grant from the Anesthesia Patient Safety Foundation (APSF) and the Foundation for Anesthesia Education and Research (FAER). The views expressed in this article are those of the authors and do not necessarily represent the official vies of APSF or FAER.

DISCLOSURE

A.F. Arriaga is the recipient of a mentored research training grant from the Anesthesia Patient Safety Foundation and the Foundation for Anesthesia Education and Research. He is the recipient of a Career Development Award from the Center for Diversity and Inclusion of the Brigham and Women's Hospital. He is a member of the Patient Safety Editorial Board for the American Society of Anesthesiologists and Question Editor for the American Board of Anesthesiology, where he receives a stipend for work that is otherwise done in a volunteer capacity. D. Szyld is the Senior Director for the Simulation Education Program of the Center for Medical Simulation. The Center for Medical Simulation provides courses and consulting to individuals and institutions in the areas of teamwork, crisis resource management, simulation-based education and debriefing. M.C.M. Pian-Smith is on the Board of Directors of both the Anesthesia Patient Safety Foundation and the Foundation for Anesthesia Education and Research. She is Adjunct Faculty for the Center for Medical Simulation. The Center for Medical Simulation provides courses and consulting to individuals and institutions in the areas of teamwork, crisis resource management, simulation-based education and debriefing.

REFERENCES

1. Gazoni FM, Amato PE, Malik ZM, et al. The impact of perioperative catastrophes on anesthesiologists: results of a national survey. Anesth Analg 2012;114(3): 596–603.
2. Charuluxananan S, Punjasawadwong Y, Suraseranivongse S, et al. The Thai Anesthesia Incidents Study (THAI Study) of anesthetic outcomes: II. Anesthetic profiles and adverse events. J Med Assoc Thai 2005;88(Suppl 7):S14–29.
3. Weiser TG, Regenbogen SE, Thompson KD, et al. An estimation of the global volume of surgery: a modelling strategy based on available data. Lancet 2008; 372(9633):139–44.
4. Weiser TG, Haynes AB, Molina G, et al. Size and distribution of the global volume of surgery in 2012. Bull World Health Organ 2016;94(3):201–209F.
5. Ziewacz JE, Arriaga AF, Bader AM, et al. Crisis checklists for the operating room: development and pilot testing. J Am Coll Surg 2011;213(2):212–7.e10.
6. Sanchez LT. Disruptive behaviors among physicians. JAMA 2014;312(21): 2209–10.
7. Arriaga AF, Sweeney RE, Clapp JT, et al. Failure to Debrief after Critical Events in Anesthesia Is Associated with Failures in Communication during the Event. Anesthesiology 2019;130(6):1039–48.
8. Zhang HF, Bo LL, Lin Y, et al. Response of Chinese Anesthesiologists to the COVID-19 Outbreak. Anesthesiology 2020;132(6):1333–8.

9. Sawyer TL, Deering S. Adaptation of the US Army's After-Action Review for simulation debriefing in healthcare. Simul Healthc 2013;8(6):388–97.

10. Brett-Fleegler M, Rudolph J, Eppich W, et al. Debriefing assessment for simulation in healthcare: development and psychometric properties. Simul Healthc 2012;7(5):288–94.

11. Mackinnon R, Gough S. What can we learn about debriefing from other high-risk/high-stakes industries? Cureus 2014;6(4):e174.

12. Heard GC, Thomas RD, Sanderson PM. In the aftermath: attitudes of anesthesiologists to supportive strategies after an unexpected intraoperative patient death. Anesth Analg 2016;122(5):1614–24.

13. Mullan PC, Kessler DO, Cheng A. Educational opportunities with postevent debriefing. JAMA 2014;312(22):2333–4.

14. Minehart RD, Rudolph J, Pian-Smith MC, et al. Improving faculty feedback to resident trainees during a simulated case: a randomized, controlled trial of an educational intervention. Anesthesiology 2014;120(1):160–71.

15. Cheng A, Nadkarni VM, Mancini MB, et al. Resuscitation education science: educational strategies to improve outcomes from cardiac arrest: a scientific statement from the American Heart Association. Circulation 2018;138(6):e82–122.

16. Dube MM, Reid J, Kaba A, et al. PEARLS for systems integration: a Modified PEARLS framework for debriefing systems-focused simulations. Simul Healthc 2019;14(5):333–42.

17. Hayes CW, Rhee A, Detsky ME, et al. Residents feel unprepared and unsupervised as leaders of cardiac arrest teams in teaching hospitals: a survey of internal medicine residents. Crit Care Med 2007;35(7):1668–72.

18. Zinns LE, O'Connell KJ, Mullan PC, et al. National survey of pediatric emergency medicine fellows on debriefing after medical resuscitations. Pediatr Emerg Care 2015;31(8):551–4.

19. Couper K, Perkins GD. Debriefing after resuscitation. Curr Opin Crit Care 2013; 19(3):188–94.

20. Kessler DO, Cheng A, Mullan PC. Debriefing in the emergency department after clinical events: a practical guide. Ann Emerg Med 2015;65(6):690–8.

21. Sawyer T, Eppich W, Brett-Fleegler M, et al. More than one way to debrief: a critical review of healthcare simulation debriefing methods. Simul Healthc 2016; 11(3):209–17.

22. Conley DM, Singer SJ, Edmondson L, et al. Effective surgical safety checklist implementation. J Am Coll Surg 2011;212(5):873–9.

23. Alidina S, Goldhaber-Fiebert SN, Hannenberg AA, et al. Factors associated with the use of cognitive aids in operating room crises: a cross-sectional study of US hospitals and ambulatory surgical centers. Implement Sci 2018;13(1):50.

24. Agarwala AV, McRichards LK, Rao V, et al. Bringing perioperative emergency manuals to your institution: a "how to" from concept to implementation in 10 steps. Jt Comm J Qual Patient Saf 2019;45(3):170–9.

25. Braithwaite J, Marks D, Taylor N. Harnessing implementation science to improve care quality and patient safety: a systematic review of targeted literature. Int J Qual Health Care 2014;26(3):321–9.

26. Rapport F, Clay-Williams R, Churruca K, et al. The struggle of translating science into action: foundational concepts of implementation science. J Eval Clin Pract 2018;24(1):117–26.

27. Salas E, Klein C, King H, et al. Debriefing medical teams: 12 evidence-based best practices and tips. Jt Comm J Qual Patient Saf 2008;34(9):518–27.

28. Voyer S, Hatala R. Debriefing and feedback: two sides of the same coin? Simul Healthc 2015;10(2):67–8.
29. van de Ridder JM, Stokking KM, McGaghie WC, et al. What is feedback in clinical education? Med Educ 2008;42(2):189–97.
30. Raemer D, Anderson M, Cheng A, et al. Research regarding debriefing as part of the learning process. Simul Healthc 2011;6(Suppl):S52–7.
31. Cheng A, Eppich W, Grant V, et al. Debriefing for technology-enhanced simulation: a systematic review and meta-analysis. Med Educ 2014;48(7):657–66.
32. Bowers C, Braun CC, Morgan BB. Team workload: its meaning and measurement. In: Brannick MT, Salas E, Prince C, editors. Team performance assessment and measurement: theory, methods, and applications. Mahwah (NJ): Lawrence Erlbaum Associates; 1997. p. 85–108.
33. Rose MR, Rose KM. Use of a surgical debriefing checklist to achieve higher value health care. Am J Med Qual 2018;33(5):514–22.
34. Haynes AB, Weiser TG, Berry WR, et al. A surgical safety checklist to reduce morbidity and mortality in a global population. N Engl J Med 2009;360(5):491–9.
35. van Klei WA, Hoff RG, van Aarnhem EE, et al. Effects of the introduction of the WHO "Surgical Safety Checklist" on in-hospital mortality: a cohort study. Ann Surg 2012;255(1):44–9.
36. Wolf FA, Way LW, Stewart L. The efficacy of medical team training: improved team performance and decreased operating room delays: a detailed analysis of 4863 cases. Ann Surg 2010;252(3):477–83 [discussion: 483–5].
37. Gillespie BM, Chaboyer W, Thalib L, et al. Effect of using a safety checklist on patient complications after surgery: a systematic review and meta-analysis. Anesthesiology 2014;120(6):1380–9.
38. Leape LL. The checklist conundrum. N Engl J Med 2014;370(11):1063–4.
39. Mitchell JT. When disaster strikes...the critical incident stress debriefing process. JEMS 1983;8(1):36–9.
40. Mitchell AM, Sakraida TJ, Kameg K. Critical incident stress debriefing: implications for best practice. Disaster Manag Response 2003;1(2):46–51.
41. Tavares W, Eppich W, Cheng A, et al. Learning conversations: an analysis of the theoretical roots and their manifestations of feedback and debriefing in medical education. Acad Med 2019;95(7):1020–5.
42. Eppich WJ, Hunt EA, Duval-Arnould JM, et al. Structuring feedback and debriefing to achieve mastery learning goals. Acad Med 2015;90(11):1501–8.
43. Eppich W, Cheng A. Promoting Excellence and Reflective Learning in Simulation (PEARLS): development and rationale for a blended approach to health care simulation debriefing. Simul Healthc 2015;10(2):106–15.
44. Bajaj K, Meguerdichian M, Thoma B, et al. The PEARLS Healthcare Debriefing Tool. Acad Med 2018;93(2):336.
45. Arriaga AF, Gawande AA, Raemer DB, et al. Pilot testing of a model for insurer-driven, large-scale multicenter simulation training for operating room teams. Ann Surg 2014;259(3):403–10.
46. Fanning RM, Gaba DM. The role of debriefing in simulation-based learning. Simul Healthc 2007;2(2):115–25.
47. Hollnagel E, Wears RL, Braithwaite J. From Safety-I to Safety-II: a White Paper. The Resilient Health Care Net: Published simultaneously by the University of Southern Denmark, University of Florida, USA, and Macquarie University, Australia. Available at: https://www.england.nhs.uk/signuptosafety/wp-content/uploads/sites/16/2015/10/safety-1-safety-2-whte-papr.pdf. Accessed May 30, 2020.

48. Tucker AL, Edmondson AC. Why hospitals don't learn from failures: organizational and psychological dynamics that inhibit system change. Calif Manag Rev 2003;45(2):55-72.

49. Brindle ME, Henrich N, Foster A, et al. Implementation of surgical debriefing programs in large health systems: an exploratory qualitative analysis. BMC Health Serv Res 2018;18(1):210.

50. Todesco J, Rasic NF, Capstick J. The effect of unanticipated perioperative death on anesthesiologists. Can J Anaesth 2010;57(4):361-7.

51. Dzau VJ, Kirch DG, Nasca TJ. To Care Is Human - Collectively Confronting the Clinician-Burnout Crisis. N Engl J Med 2018;378(4):312-4.

52. Shanafelt TD, Dyrbye LN, West CP. Addressing physician burnout: the way forward. JAMA 2017;317(9):901-2.

53. Thomas LR, Ripp JA, West CP. Charter on physician well-being. JAMA 2018; 319(15):1541-2.

54. Hu YY, Arriaga AF, Roth EM, et al. Protecting patients from an unsafe system: the etiology and recovery of intraoperative deviations in care. Ann Surg 2012;256(2): 203-10.

55. Reason JT. The human contribution: unsafe acts, accidents and heroic recoveries. Burlington (VT): Ashgate; 2008.

56. Kagee A. Concerns about the effectiveness of critical incident stress debriefing in ameliorating stress reactions. Crit Care 2002;6(1):88.

57. Mullan PC, Wuestner E, Kerr TD, et al. Implementation of an in situ qualitative debriefing tool for resuscitations. Resuscitation 2013;84(7):946-51.

58. Sandhu N, Eppich W, Mikrogianakis A, et al. Postresuscitation debriefing in the pediatric emergency department: a national needs assessment. CJEM 2014; 16(5):383-92.

59. Pittman J, Turner B, Gabbott DA. Communication between members of the cardiac arrest team–a postal survey. Resuscitation 2001;49(2):175-7.

60. Sweeney RE, Clapp JT, Arriaga AF, et al. Understanding debriefing: a qualitative study of event reconstruction at an academic medical center. Acad Med 2019; 95(7):1089-97.

61. Rudolph JW, Simon R, Raemer DB, et al. Debriefing as formative assessment: closing performance gaps in medical education. Acad Emerg Med 2008; 15(11):1010-6.

62. Pian-Smith MCM, Cooper JB. If we don't learn from our critical events, we're likely to relive them: debriefing should be the norm. Anesthesiology 2019;130(6): 867-9.

63. Rabin BA, Brownson RC, Haire-Joshu D, et al. A glossary for dissemination and implementation research in health. J Public Health Manag Pract 2008;14(2): 117-23.

64. Brownson RC, Fielding JE, Maylahn CM. Evidence-based public health: a fundamental concept for public health practice. Annu Rev Public Health 2009;30: 175-201.

65. Palinkas LA, Aarons GA, Horwitz S, et al. Mixed method designs in implementation research. Adm Policy Ment Health 2011;38(1):44-53.

66. Kirchner JE, Smith JL, Powell BJ, et al. Getting a clinical innovation into practice: an introduction to implementation strategies. Psychiatry Res 2020;283:112467.

67. Greenhalgh T, Robert G, Macfarlane F, et al. Diffusion of innovations in service organizations: systematic review and recommendations. Milbank Q 2004;82(4): 581-629.

68. Powell BJ, Waltz TJ, Chinman MJ, et al. A refined compilation of implementation strategies: results from the Expert Recommendations for Implementing Change (ERIC) project. Implement Sci 2015;10:21.
69. Damschroder LJ, Aron DC, Keith RE, et al. Fostering implementation of health services research findings into practice: a consolidated framework for advancing implementation science. Implement Sci 2009;4:50.
70. Meyers DC, Durlak JA, Wandersman A. The quality implementation framework: a synthesis of critical steps in the implementation process. Am J Community Psychol 2012;50(3–4):462–80.
71. Gagliardi AR, Marshall C, Huckson S, et al. Developing a checklist for guideline implementation planning: review and synthesis of guideline development and implementation advice. Implement Sci 2015;10:19.
72. Gillespie BM, Marshall A. Implementation of safety checklists in surgery: a realist synthesis of evidence. Implement Sci 2015;10:137.
73. Gaba DM, Fish KJ, Howard SK, et al. Crisis management in anesthesiology. Second edition. Philadelphia: Elsevier/Saunders; 2015.
74. Runciman WB, Webb RK, Klepper ID, et al. The Australian Incident Monitoring Study. Crisis management–validation of an algorithm by analysis of 2000 incident reports. Anaesth Intensive Care 1993;21(5):579–92.
75. Link MS, Berkow LC, Kudenchuk PJ, et al. Part 7: adult advanced cardiovascular life support: 2015 American Heart Association Guidelines Update for Cardiopulmonary Resuscitation and Emergency Cardiovascular Care. Circulation 2015; 132(18 Suppl 2):S444–64.
76. Moitra VK, Einav S, Thies KC, et al. Cardiac arrest in the operating room: resuscitation and management for the anesthesiologist: part 1. Anesth Analg 2018; 126(3):876–88.
77. Runciman WB, Merry AF. Crises in clinical care: an approach to management. Qual Saf Health Care 2005;14(3):156–63.
78. Hepner DL, Arriaga AF, Cooper JB, et al. Operating Room Crisis Checklists and Emergency Manuals. Anesthesiology 2017;127(2):384–92.
79. Stanford Anesthesia Cognitive Aid Group*. Emergency manual: cognitive aids for perioperative clinical events. Available at: http://emergencymanual.stanford.edu for latest version. Creative Commons BY-NC-ND. 2013 (creativecommons.org/licenses/by-nc-nd/3.0/legalcode). *Core contributors in random order: Howard SK, Chu LK, Goldhaber-Fiebert SN, Gaba DM, Harrison TK.
80. Goldhaber-Fiebert SN, Howard SK. Implementing emergency manuals: can cognitive aids help translate best practices for patient care during acute events? Anesth Analg 2013;117(5):1149–61.
81. Arriaga AF, Bader AM, Wong JM, et al. Simulation-based trial of surgical-crisis checklists. N Engl J Med 2013;368(3):246–53.
82. Emergency Manuals Implementation Collaborative. Available at: https://www.emergencymanuals.org. Accessed April 10, 2020.
83. Hannenberg AA. Cognitive aids in the management of critical events. Anesthesiol Clin 2020;38(4):789–800.
84. The Operating Room Emergency Checklist Implementation Toolkit. Available at: https://www.implementingemergencychecklists.org/. Accessed April 10, 2020.
85. Bardes JM, Biswas S, Strumwasser AM, et al. Comparison of trauma resuscitation practices by critical care anesthesiologists and non-critical care anesthesiologists. J Clin Anesth 2020;65:109890.

86. Arriaga AF, Elbardissi AW, Regenbogen SE, et al. A policy-based intervention for the reduction of communication breakdowns in inpatient surgical care: results from a Harvard surgical safety collaborative. Ann Surg 2011;253(5):849–54.

87. Lingard L, Espin S, Whyte S, et al. Communication failures in the operating room: an observational classification of recurrent types and effects. Qual Saf Health Care 2004;13(5):330–4.

88. Hu YY, Arriaga AF, Peyre SE, et al. Deconstructing intraoperative communication failures. J Surg Res 2012;177(1):37–42.

89. Greenberg CC, Regenbogen SE, Studdert DM, et al. Patterns of communication breakdowns resulting in injury to surgical patients. J Am Coll Surg 2007;204(4): 533–40.

90. Bacon AK, Morris RW, Runciman WB, et al. Crisis management during anaesthesia: recovering from a crisis. Qual Saf Health Care 2005;14(3):e25.

91. Rudolph JW, Simon R, Dufresne RL, et al. There's no such thing as "nonjudgmental" debriefing: a theory and method for debriefing with good judgment. Simul Healthc 2006;1(1):49–55.

92. Center for Medical Simulation. Available at: https://harvardmedsim.org/. Accessed April 11, 2020.

93. Delisle M, Hannenberg AA. Alternatives to high-fidelity simulation. Anesthesiol Clin 2020;38(4):761–73.

94. Cheng A, Eppich W, Kolbe M, et al. A conceptual framework for the development of debriefing skills: a journey of discovery, growth, and maturity. Simul Healthc 2020;15(1):55–60.

95. PEARLS Healthcare Debriefing Tool. Available at: https://debrief2learn.org/pearls-debriefing-tool/. Accessed April 11, 2020.

96. Rose S, Cheng A. Charge nurse facilitated clinical debriefing in the emergency department. CJEM 2018;20(5):781–5.

97. Cheng A, Grant V, Huffman J, et al. Coaching the debriefer: peer coaching to improve debriefing quality in simulation programs. Simul Healthc 2017;12(5): 319–25.

98. Wyckoff MH, Aziz K, Escobedo MB, et al. Part 13: neonatal resuscitation: 2015 American Heart Association guidelines update for cardiopulmonary resuscitation and emergency cardiovascular care. Circulation 2015;132(18 Suppl 2): S543–60.

Preparing for Mass Casualty Events

Joseph McIsaac, MD, MS, MBA, CPE[a,b],*, Brenda A. Gentz, MD[c]

KEYWORDS

- Mass casualties • CBRN • Chemical • Biological • Radiological • Nuclear
- Pandemic • Simulation exercises • SALT triage

KEY POINTS

- Mass casualty events occur regularly. Preparation reduces morbidity and mortality. Training for infrequent events, like malignant hyperthermia, is already human nature.
- The mass casualty surge is added to the usual burden of surgical disease and often requires expansion of facilities to manage successfully.
- Chemical, biological, radiological, and nuclear (CBRN) defense exposure can be a separate event or combined with traumatic injuries. CBRN events seem to be increasing.
- The Joint Commission requires twice-yearly hospital disaster exercises. Anesthesiology departments should participate at both the leadership and staff levels.
- There is a plethora of resources available for individual and team training.

INTRODUCTION

The best definition of a mass casualty incident (MCI) is any number of casualties that exceeds the resources normally available. An ability to deal with any incident depends on the number of injuries, severity of injuries, level of supplies, and support from the health care community (**Box 1**). Mass casualties can come from many sources—hurricanes, tornadoes, fires, mass shootings or stabbings, bombings, vehicle attacks, and even viral pandemics.

TYPES AND CHARACTERISTICS OF MASS CASUALTY VICTIMS

The characteristics of MCI patients are determined by the type of mass casualty event. Terrorist attacks tend to focus on soft targets where people tend to congregate, such

[a] University of Connecticut School of Medicine, Farmington, CT, USA; [b] National Disaster Medical System, US Department of Health and Human Services, Washington, DC, USA; [c] The University of Arizona College of Medicine-Tucson, Banner University Medical Center-Tucson, South Campus, 1625 North Campbell Avenue, Tucson, AZ 85719, USA
* Corresponding author. Department of Anesthesia, 263 Farmington Avenue, Farmington, CT 06030.
E-mail address: jmcisaac@uchc.edu

Anesthesiology Clin 38 (2020) 821–837
https://doi.org/10.1016/j.anclin.2020.08.008
1932-2275/20/Published by Elsevier Inc.

anesthesiology.theclinics.com

Box 1
Characteristics of a mass casualty event

- Time—sudden onset versus long time course
- Type—trauma versus infection versus chemical/radiological intoxication
- Geography—local versus regional versus national/international
- Infrastructure—degree of degradation

---

as restaurants, wedding halls, funerals, dance/concert venues, sporting events, and tourist locations. Many victims are young, and, in Israel, up to 61% were between the ages of 15 and 29, with a male predominance.[1] Earthquake survivors have a predominance of crush and extremity injuries. Combination injuries involving multiple regions of the body tend to do worse. Head injuries, in combination with another body region, such as the head/neck or torso, have the worst prognosis. Chemical and radiation injuries need decontamination but may have concomitant trauma as well. In addition, infected patients must be isolated.

DEPARTMENTAL PREPAREDNESS

Preparing for an MCI requires planning and training in 3 simultaneous areas: individual knowledge, leadership preparation, and team/department/interdepartmental skills. Templates, playbooks, and plans must be practiced, tested, and revised in an iterative manner. Having a plan that is not widely known is not the same as implementing a well-tested one. All disasters feature a lack of or degradation in infrastructure, people, or supplies. Austere conditions tend to be the rule. It is, therefore, important to consider the 4 Ss—staff, space, stuff, and systems—during planning and training (**Box 2**).

At the start of planning, a hazard vulnerability analysis (HVA) should be performed. This analysis results in a matrix of risks graded on impact and likelihood of occurrence.[2,3] All hospitals are required by the Joint Commission to perform and report an HVA. The institution's HVA can be used as the basis for a departmental HVA (**Fig. 1**).

INDIVIDUAL KNOWLEDGE

Individuals should be encouraged to develop their knowledge by ongoing reading and course participation. There are many books, chapters, Web sites, courses, and articles available (**Box 3**).[4]

Box 2
4Ss: staff, space, stuff, systems

- Staff—clinical and nonclinical
- Space—units, patient flow, staff housing, and break areas
- Stuff—logistics (medications, blood, food, sterile supplies, PPE, disposables, and medical devices [ventilators, etc.])
- Systems—infrastructure: power, water, sanitation, transportation, command and control, information and computer systems, communications, etc.

HAZARD AND VULNERABILITY ASSESSMENT TOOL
HUMAN RELATED EVENTS

EVENT	PROBABILITY	SEVERITY = (MAGNITUDE - MITIGATION)						RISK
		HUMAN IMPACT	PROPERTY IMPACT	BUSINESS IMPACT	PREPARED-NESS	INTERNAL RESPONSE	EXTERNAL RESPONSE	
	Likelihood this will occur	Possibility of death or injury	Physical losses and damages	Interuption of services	Preplanning	Time, effectivness, resouces	Community/ Mutual Aid staff and supplies	Relative threat*
SCORE	0 = N/A 1 = Low 2 = Moderate 3 = High	0 = N/A 1 = Low 2 = Moderate 3 = High	0 = N/A 1 = Low 2 = Moderate 3 = High	0 = N/A 1 = Low 2 = Moderate 3 = High	0 = N/A 1 = High 2 = Moderate 3 = Low or none	0 = N/A 1 = High 2 = Moderate 3 = Low or none	0 = N/A 1 = High 2 = Moderate 3 = Low or none	0 - 100%
Mass Casualty Incident (trauma)								0%
Mass Casualty Incident (medical/infectious)								0%
Terrorism, Biological								0%
VIP Situation								0%
Hostage Situation								0%
Civil Disturbance								0%
Missing Resident								0%
Bomb Threat								
AVERAGE								0%
*Threat increases with percentage.								0%
								0%
	0.00	0.00	0.00	0.00	0.00	0.00	0.00	0%

RISK = PROBABILITY * SEVERITY
0.00   0.00   0.00

Fig. 1. A portion of a hospital HVA template. (*From* Sample Template. FREE 9 Hazard Vulnerability Analysis Templates in PDF: MS Word: Excel. Available at: www.sampletemplates.com/business-templates/analysis/hazard-vulnerability-analysis-template.html With permission.)

IMMEDIATE RESPONDERS

It has become more widely accepted that everyone can do something to help in a time of crisis. In any disaster, there are injured casualties, first responders, and a new category of provider defined as an *immediate responder*. An immediate responder is defined as an individual who finds themselves at the incident of a scene and is able

---

Box 3
Individual training resources

- Web sites and reading lists
  - ASA Trauma and Emergency Preparedness Web site
  - Department of Health and Human Services Web site (https://www.phe.gov/preparedness/pages/default.aspx)
  - Books and handbooks
- Just-in-time training
  - PPE charts and quick references (family and CBRN) (https://www.asahq.org/about-asa/governance-and-committees/asa-committees/committee-on-trauma-and-emergency-preparedness-cotep/emergency-preparedness)
- Courses
  - Basic, core, and advanced disaster life support (https://www.ndlsf.org/)
  - Stop the Bleed (https://www.stopthebleed.org/)

to assist others. These individuals may have only minor injuries or are uninjured.[5] Through universal training and education of the citizenry, the United States has the opportunity to increase overall disaster resiliency and community outcomes following large-scale disasters. The need for local population life-saving skill training and equipping has been demonstrated and is a known, vital component of disaster risk reduction. Local communities are best positioned and suited to begin a response in the aftermath of a disaster because they have a better understanding of people, politics, resources, and local infrastructure.[5]

PREHOSPITAL MASS TRAUMA
SALT Triage

Triage refers to the evaluation and categorization of the sick or wounded when there are insufficient resources for medical care of everyone at once.[6] There are several triage systems currently embraced. The SALT triage system focuses on sorting, assessing, providing lifesaving interventions, and treatment/transport.[7] Most triage systems have at least 4 categories of patients:

- Minor emergency (green) — non–life-threatening injuries
- Delayed emergency (yellow) — urgent but can be transported in a second group
- Immediate emergency (red) — need to be transported immediately
- Expectant/dying (gray) and dead (black)

Triaging these patients correctly is critical because labeling a severely injured patient as *walking wounded* can be dangerous, but over-triage can be associated with higher mortality by clogging up wards.

STOP THE BLEED

"Uncontrolled bleeding is the number one cause of preventable death from trauma." Launched in October 2015 by the White House, Stop the Bleed is a national awareness campaign and a call to action. "Stop the Bleed is intended to cultivate grassroots efforts that encourage bystanders to become trained, equipped, and empowered to help in a bleeding emergency before professional help arrives." The Stop the Bleed campaign came out of the Hartford Consensus, which included the American College of Surgeons and other medical groups, Department of Homeland Security, the National Security Council, the Federal Bureau of Investigation, law enforcement, and fire rescue and emergency medical services (EMS). "The overarching principle of the Hartford Consensus is that no one should die from uncontrolled bleeding."[8]

Provider Safety

For medical providers, there is a tendency to rush in. Caution is warranted in that the first action in an emergency with mass casualties is to make sure that the scene is safe. Only after a scene is determined to be safe should providers at a MCI evaluate the number and severity of patients. Zones may be established within MCI scenes. The hot zone is the area of danger containing the controlled threat. The warm zone is an area that is not in direct immediate danger but has not been declared completely safe. The cold zone is the safe area for triaging, staging, and transportation of the patients.[6]

Critical Mortality

One of the most importance concepts in MCIs is *critical mortality*. That is the fraction of those individuals who are admitted to a hospital with life-threatening injuries who go on to die. A 2012 article, co-authored by Christine Gaarder, a doctor involved in the Oslo attacks, found that between 2001 and 2007 the typical critical mortality rate after a terrorist attack was between 15% and 37%.[9,10] This critical mortality has substantially improved over the past 2 decades. For example, no one died in the hospital after the Boston Marathon bombings in 2013; the hospitals in Paris saved all but 2 of the patients admitted after gunmen and suicide-bombers injured more than 400 people and killed 130 on November 13, 2015; and, finally, of the 104 admissions to the University Medical Center of Southern Nevada, after the 2017 mass shooting incident, just 4 died.[10]

Regional Hospital Systems—Hub and Spoke

Much of the success in decreasing critical mortality is due to the creation of hospital hub-and-spoke systems. This is the structuring of trauma care around expert hospitals. This occurred in Great Britain after a 2010 National Audit Office report that suggested an increased number of lives could be saved by adopting this system. In the hub-and-spoke system, critically injured patients travel to expert hospitals even if that means passing a local hospital en route.[10]

CASUALTY BEHAVIOR

Patients at the scenes often do not follow rules. In the Last Vegas shooting, the "incident scene expanded from17.5 acres to 4 square miles as survivors fled the scene and began to call 911."[11] Patients who self-evacuate may not know the location of clearing stations and present themselves at the closest local hospital. In emergencies, all forms of transportation are used—Uber, Lyft, buses, makeshift stretchers, police vehicles, ambulances, and private cars. In the Las Vegas shooting, 80% of the patients arrived by personal vehicles, cabs, or ride-sharing services from the incident—often 4 to a vehicle.[12] Rumors and misinformation can create a lot of confusion and fear during a mass casualty event. In Las Vegas, incorrect reports circulated that the area's only Level 1 trauma center was closed. There also were rumors that there were additional active shooter incidents occurring, including at one of the hospitals.[12]

COMMUNICATION

Problems with communication during a MCI are common. University of Washington Harborview Medical Center researchers "created a system that utilized a combination of text, voice and e-mail coupled with conference calls to communicate with staff in their system. Their premise behind using text messaging was the higher likelihood of successful transmission than voice calls."[13] Dr Ahmad also has been testing a system called Panacea's Cloud that is being developed as a "situational awareness operating system whose common operating picture includes communication with and tracking of patients, first responders, healthcare providers and incident commanders."[13] Communication between hospitals can be poor. "In London on July 7th, 2005, with phone networks jammed, medical students were sent running from site to site with messages on paper." A decade later, although communication has improved, Las Vegas responders still noted delays of 8 hours or longer in receiving text messages.[12]

CRISIS LEADERSHIP

The consulting firm, McKinsey, recommends that "what leaders need during a crisis is not a predefined response plan but behaviors and mindsets that will prevent them from overreacting to yesterday's developments and help them look ahead."[14] They define 5 leadership characteristic actions during a crisis. Leaders must demonstrate calm and bounded optimism. They should establish a network of teams to deal with issues at hand as well as maintaining ongoing activities. Leaders should resist the temptation to make snap decisions based on emotion. Instead, pause, anticipate events and consequences, and consult teams before a decision. Whenever possible, give decision making authority to the teams.

Leaders should maintain transparency, be honest when there is uncertainty, and give frequent updates to staff. Finally, time should be taken to express empathy toward not only the victims but also the staff, who also may be worried about themselves and their own families[15] (**Boxes 4** and **5**).

DEPARTMENTAL PLANNING AND TRAINING

Planning and preparation were best evident by the events at Bastille Day in Nice, France, on July 14, 2016, as well as the Boston Marathon bombings.[16] After earlier attacks in Paris, first responders in Nice completed an emergency event simulation involving 60 actors in May 2016. The scenario involved patients going directly to a hospital from the scene of a terrorist attack, which led to the implementation of an in-hospital medical triage process. The 2 keys points learned during the exercise were (1) the regional health system coordinated the medical and hospital resources and (2) the preparation of a hospital team dedicated to damage control resuscitation. The triage team was led by an emergency physician, a trauma surgeon, and an anesthesiologist.

The Boston Marathon bombing was the first improvised explosive device incident to cause mass casualty injuries in the United States. Bystanders pitched in to help stop bleeding and evacuate victims before responders could arrive and save lives. Crucial stabilization of trauma injuries was provided in the medical tent that was meant to accommodate up to 2500 runners and stationed near the marathon finish line. Early tourniquet use was key, and up to 26 tourniquets were place in the field. An incident command center was in place. At area hospitals, all ongoing surgeries were finished and no further elective cases were done. All 30 red-tagged patients were transported within 18 minutes and the last of the injured patients was transported from the scene within 45 minutes.[17,18]

After the World Trade Center collapsed on September 11, 2001, the US Government established the Hospital Preparedness Program to "enhance the ability of hospitals and healthcare systems to prepare for and respond to bioterror attacks...and other public health emergencies, including pandemic influenza and natural disasters."[19] The National Preparedness Goal was updated in 2015. The goal is to establish "A secure and resilient nation with the capabilities required across the whole community

---

Box 4
Crisis leadership tasks

- Demonstrate deliberate calm and bounded optimism
- Communicate effectively
- Establish a network of teams and relinquish control
- Pause to assess, then act
- Display compassion

> **Box 5**
> **Crisis communication points**
>
> - State the crisis
>   - Known, unknown
> - State what is being done (teams, logistics, staff protection)
> - State plans for future
> - Stay calm and express bounded optimism
> - Give frequent updates
> - Express empathy for patients, staff (acknowledge stress and give thanks), and families

to prevent, protect against, mitigate, respond to, and recover from the threats and hazards that pose the greatest risk."[20]

The Whole Community Approach has 6 strategic themes: (1) understand community complexity; (2) recognize community capabilities and needs; (3) foster relationships with community leaders; (4) build and maintain partnerships; (5) empower local action; and (6) leverage and strengthen social infrastructure, networks, and assets. There is recognition by the government that the local populations are often best positioned to begin response in the immediate aftermath of a disaster. The Whole Community Approach goals include prevention, protection, mitigation, response, and recovery. The implementation of this approach can be seen with the recent coronavirus outbreak.

HOSPITAL-LEVEL PREPAREDNESS

Hospitals respond to mass casualty and other disaster incidents by setting up their Hospital Incident Command System Command Center and implementing their Incident Response Plan.[21] Anesthesiology departmental leadership (chair, vice, chair, and clinical managers) should be familiar with the system. Federal Emergency Management Agency offers a series of free online courses for familiarization with the system (IC100, Introduction to the Incident Response System, through IC 800, Introduction to the National Response Framework, https://training.fema.gov/is/).

The ASA has a Guide to Anesthesia Department Administration, offering an easy to read guide for the chair to implement a department preparedness plan (https://www.asahq.org/quality-and-practice-management/quality-improvement/qmda-regulatory-toolkit/guide-to-anesthesia-department-administration/defining-mass-casualty-events-and-natural-disasters). The older but more complete version can be found at https://www.asahq.org/about-asa/governance-and-committees/asa-committees/committee-on-trauma-and-emergency-preparedness-cotep/emergency-preparedness.

The ASA has also developed checklists for operating room management during mass casualties, operating room power failures, and family preparedness (**Fig. 2**) (https://www.asahq.org/about-asa/governance-and-committees/asa-committees/committee-on-trauma-and-emergency-preparedness-cotep/emergency-preparedness).

Exercise and Simulation

Resources for conducting simulations at whole hospital level and departmental level are available that can help to provide vicarious experience to both leaders and staff.[22] These can take the form of tabletop exercises for leaders, online simulations, and hands-on unit/interunit training.[23] Anesthesiologists can participate in hospital

Objective

To be able to manage the flow of patient care in the OR's during a mass casualty situation.

Steps (Indicate date and time for each item)

☐ Refer to facility's Operation's Manual

Open up appropriate annex

☐ **Activate call-in tree**

Assign an individual to activate. Use clerical personnel or automatic paging system, if available

☐ Assess status of operating rooms

Determine staffing of OR's 0-2, 2-12 and 12-24 hours. Hold elective cases.

☐ **Alert current OR's**

Finish current surgical procedures as soon as possible and prepare to receive trauma

☐ Assign staff

Set up for trauma/emergency cases

☐ **Anesthesia Coordinator should become OR Medical Director**

Work with OR Nursing Manager to facilitate communication and coordination of staff and facilities

☐ **Report OR status to Hospital Command Center (HCC)**

Enter telephone, email address of HCC

☐ Ensure adequate supplies

Coordinate with anesthesia techs/supply personnel to ensure adequate supplies of fluids, medications, disposables, other

☐ Contact PACU

Accelerate transfer of patients to floors/ICU's in preparation for high volume of cases

☐ Anesthesiologist should act as liaison in Emergency Department (ED)

Send an experienced practitioner to the ED to act as a liaison (your eyes & ears) and keep communications open to Anesthesia Coordinator

☐ Consider assembly of Stat Teams

Combination of anesthesia, surgical, nursing, respiratory personnel to triage, as needed

☐ HAZMET/WMD event

Review special personal protective procedures, such as DECON & isolation techniques. Consider if part of the OR or hallways should be considered "hot" or should have ventilation altered. Good resources include CHEMM/REMM websites

Fig. 2. Operating room procedures for mass casualty management step by step. (*From* American Society of Anesthesiologists. Emergency Preparedness. Available at: https://www.asahq.org/about-asa/governance-and-committees/asa-committees/committee-on-trauma-and-emergency-preparedness-cotep/emergency-preparedness With permission.)

exercises as a whole department or in as small as a single operating room, depending on resources. Lessons learned from small exercises can be disseminated to the entire department.[24]

Secondary Attacks

Hospitals may be targets of primary or secondary attacks (eg, Mumbai, India, 2008). Be aware that if shootings or other incidents occur within hospitals, the hospital itself can be declared a hot zone. Security personnel should maintain clear vehicle entry points and monitor access to the emergency department (ED). All entrances to the facility will need to be controlled. "Ideally, law enforcement should be present to support hospital security at the entrance and provide traffic control."[11] Police have to clear staff prior to allowing them to enter and/or return to work. These lockdowns can control access to elevators, critical equipment, and operating rooms.[18]

Hospital Organization During Mass Casualty Events

Although patients may have been triaged in the field, it may be appropriate to perform a second triage upon arrival to determine if patients have deteriorated. A zone should be set up in the ED where the walking wounded may be monitored. There are patients who arrive who either leave may on their own or go to another institution. Try to maintain unidirectional flow in the ED (ie, the patients should not return to the ED once they have been taken to radiology, the operating room, or other areas). During a mass casualty event, failure of electronic systems may require staff to revert to paper. Similarly, it is important to be able to back up electronic registration systems in the event that the wireless networks are overwhelmed. Also, it should be ensured that there is an adequate supply of paper triage tags and/or paper charts.[11]

Practical lessons from past MCIs include

- Bringing essential assets to the ground floor, including carts, wheelchairs, personnel, and, designated disaster supplies
- Popping up heads on gurneys so patients are not placed on them backwards[11,25]
- Using portable monitors
- Before patients arrive, if possible, clearing the ED
- Discharging as many preexisting patients as possible
- Cohorting patients requiring additional work-up
- Transporting admitted patients to their designated floors or intensive care units (ICUs)
- Identifing areas that may be used for expanded ED, floor, and/or ICU space

Patient Identification

Patients may arrive without identification or anyone who can identify them. "In Las Vegas, many patients attended the concert wearing only their entrance wristbands, cell phones and small amounts of cash."[11] Some hospital systems like to reassign trauma patients to their correct names as quickly as possible. During MCIs, this can increase confusion, especially if there are multiple family members with the same last name or even senior and juniors. One suggestion is to change the unidentified name to that of a state, town, city, or color so as to create a more obvious difference between patients. Complicating identification further, during MCIs, patients may have consumed variable amounts of alcohol. Identifying characteristics, such as body art and piercings, may be helpful in matching unconscious patients with their family members.[11] During the Las Vegas shooting, a need was recognized for a centralized data hub, where descriptions of identified patients in a massive emergency could be uploaded and information accessed by all area hospitals.[26]

EARLY INTERVENTIONS

Because patients can deteriorate while waiting for care, the early placement of intravenous access can be critical. One of the actions that the Sunrise Hospital ED physicians felt saved lives was placing intravenous access early in the patients who presented from the Las Vegas mass shooting. They made sure that all patients had 14-gauge to 18-gauge intravenous catheters ready for the moment that they might decompensate.[25] EMS providers may be able to assist in placing intraosseous infusions during the early response to the incident.[27] Consider pairing a nurse, a medical student, or another provider with each patient until there is a handoff to the operating room, ICU, or floor. This is someone who knows about the patient's medical history and the interventions that have been completed and can monitor for changes in condition.[11] Provide focused care delivery when possible. This includes controlling critical bleeding with tourniquets to convert patients from red to yellow. Plan to intubate patients who are unable to speak. Insert chest tubes, if needed. Consider intraosseous access to save time. Follow mental status changes and monitor motor examinatino changes. Keep the patients warm and continually reassess.[28]

SUPPORT SERVICES

Consider ordering a trauma panel for all patients, but beware of saturating the laboratory with unnecessary studies and blood bank with many type/screens that may not be needed.[28] "Dedicate pharmacy personnel and resources in the ED to ensure adequate medication supplies. Automated medication dispensing stations may be unable to keep up with the volume of needed medications."[11,25] Dedicate a respiratory therapist for intubation support in the ED. Consider prepackaged disaster intubation or critical care supply packs for bedside use.[11] In extreme situations, ventilator splitting can be considered. If there are 2 people who are approximately the same size and tidal volume, it is possible to double the tidal volume and connect them via Y tubing on 1 ventilator. But is this practical? Although this idea was discussed in the event of a serious ventilator shortage during the coronavirus disease (COVID-19) outbreak, it tends to be not practical because of the differences in cohort stage of disease, overall pulmonary resistance, and compliance issues.[25] Radiology can be a bottleneck on the way to the ICU or operating room. Consider having the radiologist read the radiographs as they are taken with a portable machine. Point-of-care ultrasound can be a helpful rapid triage tool when available at the bedside and time allows.

Damage Control Surgery

Surgeons do the minimum necessary surgery to save a patient's life. "Damage control surgery involves performing only necessary amounts of surgery to control bleeding, remove nonviable tissue, stabilize fractures and restore extremity perfusion."[29] The first priority for the OR is unstable patients with isolated abdominal injuries, followed by patients with chest injuries. Neurologic injuries are addressed on a case-by-case basis. Vascular injury with threatened limb should be a high priority as well. Most extremity injuries (uncomplicated fractures and soft tissue injury without vascular compromise) can be deferred for at least a few hours.

STAFFING ISSUES

In the London Bridge incident, many on-call staff found out an attack was under way via Twitter or WhatsApp and set out unprompted.[10] It is not beneficial for everyone to respond in the first wave. Do not call in all personnel at the onset of the incident. Providers will become fatigued and need relief. Ask some to come in at a later time to relieve staff who cared for the initial influx of patients. Staff members who may need to be called in include environmental services, materials management, administrative services (scribes), volunteers, and ancillary personnel (laboratory, radiology, and pharmacy technicians and respiratory therapists).[11] A system for calling in staff should be a part of the institutional disaster plan.

Surge Discharge

During critical events, it is important to have hospitalists and intensivist do rounds and assess inpatients for potential surge discharge.[11] It also is important as the events wind down to identify a single location where patients may wait (eg, discharge lounge) while other arrangements are made if the incident delays their ability to leave the hospital so that bed availability is maximized. "At Sunrise Hospital, they allowed released patients to wait in the auditorium until other arrangements could be made. University Medical Center arranged transportation to a designated pick-up location."[11]

Do Not Return to a Normal Operating Room Schedule Too Quickly

After the surge subsides, hospitals try to return to their normal schedules as soon as possible. A major incident can be declared over too soon. After the 2017 Manchester Arena bombing, "some hospitals in Manchester (England) restarted elective surgeries a few hours after the bombing yet in the following days, the injured required 139 hours of additional theater time - about two normal weeks' worth of surgery."[10] "Over 350 hours of extra surgery were required in the week after the terrorist attack in Manchester" (personal communication from Greater Manchester Trauma Network).[30] There is a recovery period where the demand for services will slowly return to normal and the demand will have been met.

NONTRADITIONAL ROLES OF ANESTHESIOLOGISTS

During a crisis, anesthesiologists are well suited to assume other roles in hospital settings. In the EDs, anesthesiologists can re-evaluate and reassign triage levels and update teams on status changes. They can assist with operating room staffing requirements and create teams that can provide around-the-clock coverage for intubation and line (arterial and central) placement. Anesthesiologists may be able to provide critical care services in the ICU. As operating room managers and directors, anesthesiologists can enable information sharing and assessment. This can include handoffs, where the anesthesiologist is acting as a bridge between the ED, operating room, and the ICU. They may be able to assist with collecting patient information, patient identification, and providing family assistance. They also may provide assistance with pain management.[27]

NONTRADITIONAL ROLES

Physicians and surgeons may want to help but may not know how. In Las Vegas, "pediatric and obstetric surgeons assisted general surgery by performing 'opening' of abdominal cases or scrubbing in to replace scrub nurses."[27] Pediatric emergency staff may be able to provide care for ambulatory adult patients in the ED. "Non-clinicians assisted with bleeding control as patients were being triaged, transported patients throughout the hospital, rapidly turned overs room and participated in fatality management activities in response to the Las Vegas no-notice incident."[27] If the hospital or site becomes overwhelmed, it may be possible that triage must be turned over to nonphysician colleagues.

SPECIAL POPULATIONS: PEDIATRICS AND OBSTETRICS

Children and pregnant women usually are a significant proportion of the casualty burden and often present to the closest hospital, regardless of whether it normally cares for these patients. Therefore, it is critical that all providers and institutions make provisions for receiving children and parturients who may be casualties or accompany casualties. Adequate supplies of pediatric equipment and the ability to do both vaginal and cesarean deliveries should be part of preparation and planning. Staff should have ready references and access to guidelines for special populations.[31,32]

NUCLEAR/RADIOLOGICAL EVENTS

Radiological exposure consists of acute radiation syndrome (ARS), radiation burns, and internal contamination.[33] In such an incident, all casualties should be decontaminated externally to limit exposure. The ARS should be treated according to the dose received.[34] Internal contamination is treated with specific therapies dependent on the radionuclide ingested.[35,36] Alternatively, oral activated charcoal has been advocated to remove gastrointestinal contamination. Surgeries should be limited to immediate trauma care and delayed, when possible, until immune function returns (**Fig. 3**).

CHEMICAL EVENTS

Chemical injuries can be categorized as inhalational injury, skin chemical burns, and intoxification syndromes. They can be a result of a local event, a large-scale industrial accident, or a chemical weapon. There often is associated conventional traumatic injury. Patients should be decontaminated of any persistent agents while responders should wear appropriate personal protective equipment (PPE). Lifesaving interventions like respiratory support should not be delayed for decontamination, but decontamination limits the injury. Toxic syndromes, like cyanide and nerve agent poisoning, should be treated with specific antidotes, when available.[37]

BIOLOGICAL EVENTS

The classic biological event is an epidemic or pandemic. Influenza had been a common model until the current coronavirus (severe acute respiratory syndrome coronavirus 2 and COVID-19) pandemic that originated in China and spread throughout the world in a matter of months. Epidemics are not unprecedented and have been a source of mass casualties since the earliest recorded history. Smallpox, plague, influenza, and viral fevers, such as Ebola, are a few examples. Deliberate release of biological agents, bioterrorism, and biological warfare, are 2 additional sources of mass casualty generation.[38]

TABLE XII. PRINCIPAL THERAPEUTIC MEASURES FOR ACUTE RADIATION SYNDROME ACCORDING TO DEGREE OF SEVERITY

Whole body dose (Gy)	1–2	2–4	4–6	6–8	>8
Degree of severity of ARS	Mild	Moderate	Severe	Very severe	Lethal
Medical management and treatment	Ouapatient observation for maximum of one month	Hospitalization			
		Isolation, as early as possible			
		G-CSF or GM-CSF as early as possible (or within the first week)		IL-3 and GM-CSF	
		Antibiotics of broad spectrum activity (from the end of the latent period) Antifungal and antiviral preparations (when necessary)			
		Blood components transfusion: platelets, erythrocytes (when necessary)			
			Complete parenteral nutrition (first week) Metabolism correction, detoxication (when necessary)		
			Plasmapheresis (second or third week) Prophylaxis of disseminated intravascular coagulation (second week)		
				HLA-identical allogene BMT (first week)	Symptomatic therapy only

Fig. 3. ARS. BMT, bone marrow transplantation; G-CSF, granulocyte-colony stimulating factor; GM-CSF, granulocyte macrophage-colony stimulating factor; IL-3, interleukin 3. (*From* "Diagnosis and Treatment of Radiation Injuries." IAEA, No. 2, 1998. Safety Reports Series. Pg. 20; with permission. Available at: https://www-pub.iaea.org/MTCD/publications/PDF/P040_scr.pdf.)

There are 2 main principles for containment and protection of caregivers: isolation and barrier protection using PPE. The most common PPE consists of barrier protection (gloves, face shield, and gown) plus respiratory protection (surgical mask, N95, N100, or powered air-purifying respirators). The highest levels of respiratory protection are needed for aerosol-generating procedures, like intubation, and for airborne transmissible diseases, like measles. Isolation, especially in a negative pressure environment, prevents the further spread of disease from infected individuals. Quarantine isolates potentially infected individuals until they are proved ill or disease-free.[39] It is critical to stockpile PPE and disinfectants in advance. The COVID-19 pandemic demonstrated the massive need for PPE. Contingency plans also should be made for conservation, recycling, and reprocessing of PPE. Planning should also be done to facilitate routine surgical care for patients who are infected or suspected of infection. This includes trauma and nonsurgical procedures done under anesthesia.

EVACUATION AND INTERFACILITY TRANSFERS

During an MCI, trauma centers may not be able to accept transfers of patients whose injuries are within their usual level of care. The emergency physician may need to make plans to stabilize and manage high-acuity patients who normally would be immediately transferred to a trauma center. Tracking large numbers of patients who must be transferred during an MCI can be difficult. "During the Santa Rosa fire, patients had to emergently transferred out of the hospitals, they took photos of the patient's wristbands with smartphones because they didn't have time to copy and write down the information from the patient's wrist bands."[26]

RESILIENCE AND RECOVERY: POSTEVENT CONSIDERATIONS

"In 2011, the deadliest single tornado recorded in the U.S. since recordkeeping began in 1950 struck Joplin, Missouri. It destroyed 7000 homes, resulted in 162 fatalities, and over 1000 individuals were injured, and cost an estimated $3 billion in insured losses."[13] "In a retrospective analysis, it was concluded that the high fatality rate was due to the intensity of the tornado and the large size of the damage area, but also factors such as ignoring the warning sirens, having less than 15 minutes to seek shelter, structural weakness in homes and disproportionate damage to a hospital and area business where more people were gathered."[13,40] A component of delayed recognition of a rare fungal infection also contributed to late deaths—zygomycosis, which is a fungal infection occurred when dirt becomes embedded under the skin, resulting in patients succumbing to a widely disseminated infections.[41]

FOLLOW-UP: TRANSMITTED DISEASES, OPHTHALMIC, AUDITORY, AND PSYCHOLOGICAL INJURIES

Patients can be placed at risk of blood-borne virus infection after MCIs and need counseling, postexposure prophylaxis, and follow-up health screens."[30,42] Human tissue can be transferred from shrapnel or contaminated knives; thus, postexposure prophylaxis should be considered. For example, in the Boston Marathon bombing, all of the patients seen with evidence for external injury were screened for evidence of preexisting hepatitis B antibodies and treated accordingly. In addition, estimates of upward of more than 100 patients out of 281 in Boston have been reported to have sustained tympanic membrane or inner ear damage.[18]

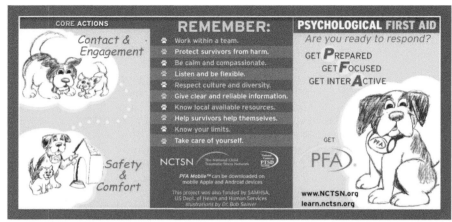

Psychological First Aid Wallet Card (back)

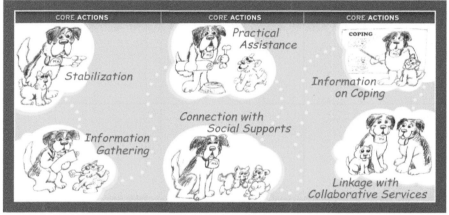

Psychological First Aid Wallet Card (front)

Fig. 4. Psychological first aid wallet card (front and back). (*From* Psychological First Aid Wallet Card. NCTSN. 2016, Available at: https://www.nctsn.org/resources/psychological-first-aid-pfa-wallet-card; with permission.)

PSYCHOLOGICAL PREPAREDNESS/BEREAVEMENT/DEBRIEFING

"One doctor involved in the Manchester attacks still hears the voices of injured parents who awoke screaming for lost children."[10] Providing psychological support for victims and health care providers of MCIs is crucial. Posttraumatic stress disorder is not uncommon. As an ED physician involved in the Santa Rosa fires aptly stated, "You never know how you are going to react until it comes your way."[26] Psychological first aid for everyone involved is a must (**Fig. 4**). After an MCI, it is important to conduct debriefings to evaluate the aspects that were handled well and those systems that should be improved. It is important to admit mistakes. Hospitals need to have an open and honest attitude toward error.

SUMMARY

Mass casualty events occur more often than we would like. Their frequency seems to be increasing. Just as the rare malignant hyperthermia case is trained for, mass casualty training should be integrated into routine preparation. Being prepared will save lives and reduce suffering.

DISCLOSURE

The authors have nothing to disclose.

REFERENCES

1. Peleg K, Aharonson-Daniel L, Michael M, et al. Patterns of Injury in Hospitalized Terrorist Victims. Am J Emerg Med 2003;21(4):258–62.
2. Hazard Vulnerability/Risk Assessment. ASPR TRACIE. Available at: asprtracie.hhs.gov/technical-resources/3/hazard-vulnerability-risk-assessment/1. Accessed July 21, 2020.
3. FREE 9 Hazard Vulnerability Analysis Templates in PDF: MS Word: Excel. FREE 9 Hazard Vulnerability Analysis Templates in PDF | MS Word | Excel. 2020. Available at: www.sampletemplates.com/business-templates/analysis/hazard-vulnerability-analysis-template.html. Accessed July 21, 2020.
4. Available at: https://www.asahq.org/about-asa/governance-and-committees/asa-committees/committee-on-trauma-and-emergency-preparedness-cotep. Accessed July 21, 2020.
5. Harris C, McCarthy K, Liu E, et al. Expanding Understanding of Response Roles: An Examination of Immediate and First Responders in the United States. Int J Environ Res Public Health 2018;15(3):534.
6. Edgerly D. The Basics of Mass Casualty Triage. JEMS 2019;41(5). Available at: www.jems.com/2016/05/01/the-basics-of-mass-casualty-triage/.
7. SALT Mass Casualty Triage. National Disaster Life Support Foundation (NDLSF). 2020. Available at: www.ndlsf.org/salt/. Accessed July 21, 2020.
8. Stop the Bleed. Department of Public Safety, University of Utah. Available at: dps.utah.edu/stopthebleed/. Accessed July 21, 2020.
9. Gaarder C, Jorgensen J, Kolstadbraaten KM, et al. The twin terrorist attacks in Norway on July 22, 2011: the trauma center response. J Trauma Acute Care Surg 2012;73(1):269–75.
10. Trauma Medicine Has Learned Lessons from the Battlefield. The Economist, The Economist Newspaper 2017. Available at: www.economist.com/international/2017/10/12/trauma-medicine-has-learned-lessons-from-the-battlefield. Accessed April 22 2020.
11. No-Notice Incidents: Triage, Hospital Intake, and Throughput. Tracie. 2018. Available at: https://files.asprtracie.hhs.gov/documents/no-notice-incidents-triage-intake-throughput.pdf. Accessed April 25, 2020.
12. No-Notice Incidents: Non-Trauma Hospital Considerations. Tracie. 2018. Available at: https://files.asprtracie.hhs.gov/documents/no-notice-incidents-non-trauma-hospital-considerations.pdf. Accessed April 24, 2020.
13. Ahmad S. Mass Casualty Incident Management. Mo Med 2018;115(5):451–5.
14. D'Auria G and De Smet A. Leadership in a crisis: responding to the coronavirus outbreak and future challenges. McKinsey & Company. Available at: www.mckinsey.com/business-functions/organization/our-insights/leadership-in-a-crisis-responding-to-the-coronavirus-outbreak-and-future-challenges. Accessed July 1, 2020.
15. McNulty EJ, Marcus L. Are You Leading Through the Crisis … or Managing the Response? Harvard Business Review 2020. Available at: hbr.org/2020/03/are-you-leading-through-the-crisis-or-managing-the-response.

16. Lord D. France Terror Attack: What Is Bastille Day? Ajc, Cox Media Group National Content Desk. 2016. Available at: www.ajc.com/news/national/france-terror-attack-what-bastille-day/dyivVC3SptQIddE0AXjUWI/. Accessed April 22, 2020.
17. Biddinger PD, Baggish A, Harrington L, et al. Be prepared–the Boston Marathon and mass-casualty events. N Engl J Med 2013;368(21):1958–60.
18. Gates JD, Arabian S, Biddinger P, et al. The Initial Response to the Boston Marathon Bombing: Lessons Learned to Prepare for the next Disaster. Ann Surg 2017; 260(6):960. Available at: www.ncbi.nlm.nih.gov/pmc/articles/PMC5531449/.
19. Hospitals Rising to the Challenge: The First Five Years of the U.S. Hospital Preparedness Program and Priorities Going Forward. UPMC Biosecurity. 2009. Available at: https://www.centerforhealthsecurity.org/our-work/pubs_archive/pubs-pdfs/2009/2009-04-16-hppreport.pdf. Accessed April 26, 2020.
20. National Preparedness Goal. Fema.gov. 2015. Available at: https://www.fema.gov/media-library-data/1443799615171-aae90be55041740f97e8532fc680d40/National_Preparedness_Goal_2nd_Edition.pdf. Accessed April 26, 2020.
21. Hospital Incident Command System – Current Guidebook and Appendices. EMSA, State of California. 2016. Available at: emsa.ca.gov/disaster-medical-services-division-hospital-incident-command-system/. Accessed July 21, 2020.
22. Hospital Surge Evaluation Tool. Phe.gov. 2017. Available at: www.phe.gov/preparedness/planning/hpp/surge/pages/default.aspx. Accessed July 21, 2020.
23. Free Joint Commission Emergency Management Training for Hospitals. Emergency Preparedness. 2017. Available at: www.calhospitalprepare.org/post/free-joint-commission-emergency-management-training-hospitals. Accessed July 21, 2020.
24. Drills & Exercises. Emergency Preparedness. 2017. Available at: www.calhospitalprepare.org/exercises. Accessed July 21, 2020.
25. Menes K. How One Las Vegas ED Saved Hundreds of Lives After the Worst Mass Shooting in U.S. History. Emergency Physicians Monthly. 2017. Available at: epmonthly.com/article/not-heroes-wear-capes-one-las-vegas-ed-saved-hundreds-lives-worst-mass-shooting-u-s-history/. Accessed April 25, 2020.
26. Ibarra AB. Hospitals' Best-Laid Plans Upended By Disaster. Kaiser Health News 2018. Available at: khn.org/news/hospitals-best-laid-plans-upended-by-disaster/. Accessed April 25, 2020.
27. No-Notice Incidents: Expanding Traditional Roles to Address Patient Surge. Tracie. 2018. Available at: https://files.asprtracie.hhs.gov/documents/no-notice-incidents-expanding-traditional-roles.pdf. Accessed April 25, 2020.
28. No-Notice Incidents: Trauma Surgery Adaptations and Lessons. Tracie. 2018. Available at: https://files.asprtracie.hhs.gov/documents/no-notice-incidents-trauma-surgery-adaptations-and-lessons.pdf. Accessed April 24, 2020.
29. Elster EA, Butler FK, Rasmussen TE. Implications of Combat Casualty Care for Mass Casualty Events. JAMA 2013;310(5):475. pubmed.ncbi.nlm.nih.gov/23925612/.
30. Moran CG, Webb C, Brohi K, et al. Lessons in Planning From Mass Casualty Events in UK. BMJ (Clin Res Ed) 2017. pubmed.ncbi.nlm.nih.gov/29070605/.
31. Pediatric Anesthesia. OpenAnesthesia. Available at: www.openanesthesia.org/pediatric_anesthesia_anesthesia_text/. Accessed July 21, 2020.
32. Cognitive Aids in Medicine. OB Anesthesia Emergency Manual. Cognitive Aids in Medicine. 2020. Available at: med.stanford.edu/cogaids/obanesem.html. Accessed July 21, 2020.
33. Radiation Emergency Medical Management, REMM. Available at: www.remm.nlm.gov/. Accessed July 21, 2020.

34. Time Phases of Acute Radiation Syndrome (ARS). Radiation Emergency Medical Management, REMM. 2020. Available at: www.remm.nlm.gov/ars_timephases1. htm. Accessed July 21, 2020.

35. HHS/ASPR. A decision makers guide: medical planning and response for a nuclear detonation. 2nd edition. Washington, DC: Assistant Secretary for Preparedness and Response, Department of Health and Human Services;; 2017. p. 38.

36. International Atomic Energy Agency. Diagnosis and Treatment of Radiation Injuries. Safety Reports Series No. 2. Vienna (Austria): IAEA; 1998.

37. McIsaac J, McQueen K, Kucik C. Essentials of disaster anesthesia. Cambridge (UK): Cambridge University Press; 2020.

38. Bioterrorism. Phe.gov. 2011. Available at: www.phe.gov/emergency/bioterrorism/Pages/default.aspx. Accessed July 21, 2020.

39. Available at: https://www.asahq.org/about-asa/governance-and-committees/asa-committees/committee-on-occupational-health/ebola-information. Accessed July 21, 2020.

40. Paul BK, Stimers M. Exploring probable reasons for record fatalities: the case of 2011 Joplin, Missouri, Tornado. Nat Hazards 2012;64:1511–26.

41. "Latest Joplin Victims Had Rare Fungus from Dirt." NBCNews.com, NBCUniversal News Group. 2011. Available at: www.nbcnews.com/id/43358247/ns/health-infectious_diseases/t/latest-joplin-victims-had-rare-fungus-dirt/. Accessed July 21, 2020.

42. England, Public Health. "Bloodborne Viruses: Managing Severe Serial Penetrating Injuries." GOV.UK. 2017. Available at: www.gov.uk/government/publications/bloodborne-viruses-managing-severe-serial-penetrating-injuries. Accessed July 21, 2020.

Obstetric Hemorrhage

Joy L. Hawkins, MD

KEYWORDS

- Maternal morbidity • Postpartum hemorrhage • Massive transfusion
- Abnormal placentation • Uterine atony

KEY POINTS

- More than half the cases of maternal mortality and severe morbidity due to hemorrhage are preventable, and in those cases diagnosis was delayed, transfusion was started late, and communication was poor between teams. All hospitals with obstetric services should have postpartum hemorrhage and massive transfusion protocols in place as well as regular training and simulation drills to ensure unit preparedness.
- Know the oxytocic medications: their dose, route of administration, and side effects. Understand obstetric techniques such as uterine tamponade, uterine compression sutures, and uterine devascularization procedures used to manage obstetric hemorrhage.
- Changes in vital signs are generally not seen until a parturient has lost up to 25% or 1500 mL of her blood volume, so quantitative estimations of blood loss are recommended. Transfuse blood products 1 packed red blood cells: 1 fresh frozen plasma: 1 platelet unit as much as possible and follow fibrinogen levels as well as other laboratory studies. Keep fibrinogen levels greater than 300 mg/dL using cryoprecipitate. Point-of-care testing including thromboelastography and rotational thromboelastometry has benefit. Consider cell salvage if available. A closed circuit can be established for patients of Jehovah's Witness faith.
- Use tranexamic acid as early as possible and within 3 hours of delivery. Recombinant Factor VIIa should be used with caution due to a 5% risk of thrombotic complications. Little is known about other factor concentrates in the setting of postpartum hemorrhage.
- Consult with an interventional radiologist if available in your facility. For hemodynamically stable patients, arterial embolization can be an effective treatment for persistent bleeding. As a last resort during uncontrolled hemorrhage, consider use of the Resuscitative Endovascular Balloon Occlusion of the Aorta (REBOA) device and damage-control surgery with resuscitation in the intensive care unit.

INTRODUCTION

Postpartum hemorrhage is defined as cumulative blood loss ≥1000 mL or bleeding associated with signs/symptoms of hypovolemia within 24 hours of birth, regardless of delivery route.[1] The Centers for Disease Control and Prevention report on pregnancy-related deaths in the United States found that approximately 700 women

University of Colorado School of Medicine, 12631 East 17th Avenue, Mail Stop 8202, Aurora, CO 80045, USA
E-mail address: Joy.Hawkins@cuanschutz.edu

Anesthesiology Clin 38 (2020) 839–858
https://doi.org/10.1016/j.anclin.2020.08.010
1932-2275/20/© 2020 Elsevier Inc. All rights reserved.
anesthesiology.theclinics.com

die annually from pregnancy-related complications, and hemorrhage accounted for 11.2% of their deaths.[2] Hemorrhage remains the most common cause of maternal mortality worldwide.[3] However, mortality only represents the tip of the iceberg as compared with tracking near-misses and severe morbidity as a clinical outcome. A study looking at 115,502 women at 25 hospitals in the Maternal-Fetal Medicine Units (MFMU) Network found that severe maternal morbidity occurred in 2.9 of 1000 births, and that severe postpartum hemorrhage was responsible for approximately half of the cases.[4] In their study women were classified as having severe maternal morbidity according to a scoring system that takes into account the occurrence of red blood cell (RBC) transfusion (more than 3 units), intubation, unanticipated surgical intervention, organ failure, and intensive care unit admission. In their population, severe morbidity was 50 times more common than maternal mortality. Anesthesiologists will always be involved at some point in the management and resuscitation of severe obstetric hemorrhage and can make a difference in improving these outcomes.

EPIDEMIOLOGY

The American Society of Anesthesiologists' (ASA) Closed Claims Project reviewed closed anesthesia malpractice claims related to hemorrhage from all causes and found that obstetric patients accounted for the largest group of claims (30%).[5] Common contributing factors in these cases were delayed diagnosis of severe hemorrhage, delayed transfusion, and poor team communication. Many series have found a high level of preventability in maternal deaths due to hemorrhage.[6] How can we do better? All obstetric facilities should have a standardized hospital-wide process in place for management of obstetric hemorrhage.[1] These bundles of standardized, multistage evaluation and response protocols have been associated with earlier intervention and resolution of maternal hemorrhage. For example, the National Partnership for Maternal Safety Consensus Bundle on Obstetric Hemorrhage was developed by a multidisciplinary team of obstetricians, maternal-fetal medicine specialists, midwives, anesthesiologists, and labor and delivery (L&D) nurses.[7] The bundle provides a system to implement key elements in 4 categories: (1) unit readiness to respond to a maternal hemorrhage, (2) recognition and prevention measures to apply to all obstetric patients, (3) a multidisciplinary response to excessive maternal bleeding in an individual patient, and (4) a post-event quality improvement process to identify systems issues and improve responsiveness. All hospitals with an obstetric service should adopt such a system.

Which mothers are most at risk of significant hemorrhage? A review of 8.5 million deliveries in the National Inpatient Sample from 1999 to 2008 found the incidence of postpartum hemorrhage doubled over the time reviewed to 4.2 per 1000 deliveries.[8] Significant risk factors for severe hemorrhage included placenta previa or abruption (adjusted odds ratio [aOR] 7.0), preeclampsia (aOR 3.1), amnionitis (aOR 2.9) and multiple pregnancy (aOR 2.8) (**Table 1**). A similar review of deliveries in New York State found the risk factors most strongly associated with massive transfusion (defined as requiring 10 or more units of blood) included abnormal placentation such as placenta previa, accreta, increta, or percreta (aOR 18.5), placental abruption (aOR 14.6), severe preeclampsia (aOR 10.4) and intrauterine fetal demise (aOR 5.5).[9] Women with 1 or more of these risk factors should be informed of their possibility of hemorrhage and transfusion, deliver in a hospital with resources to manage massive transfusion, and have adequate intravenous access and type and cross-matched blood available before delivery. However, many women without risk factors experience postpartum

Table 1
Risk factors for severe obstetric hemorrhage

Obstetric Condition	Adjusted Odds Ratio
Abnormal placentation (eg, accreta spectrum)[9,42]	18.5
Placental abruption[9]	14.6
Severe preeclampsia[8,9]	3.1/10.4
Placenta previa or abruption[8]	7.0
Intrauterine fetal demise[9]	5.5
Amnionitis[8]	2.9
Multiple pregnancy[8]	2.8

Data from Refs.[8,9,42]

hemorrhage, and most women with risk factors do not experience significant hemorrhage. Diligent surveillance of all patients is needed.

MANAGEMENT STRATEGIES UNIQUE TO PERIPARTUM HEMORRHAGE

The American College of Obstetricians and Gynecologists (ACOG) has a Patient Safety Checklist for postpartum hemorrhage within their Safe Motherhood Initiative to guide management during maternal hemorrhage[10] (**Fig. 1**). It describes a systematic approach, escalating care at 500, 1000, and 1500 mL estimated blood loss (EBL). Escalation of care includes calling the anesthesiology team for help by the time blood loss reaches 1000 mL, and initiating the massive transfusion protocol when EBL reaches 1500 mL. Unfortunately, caregivers on L&D (including nurses, obstetricians, midwives, and anesthesiologists) are not accurate when visually estimating blood loss during delivery, and postpartum blood loss is significantly underestimated. This leads to delayed diagnosis and delayed transfusion because most peripartum women are young and healthy and can compensate for hypovolemia for an extended time.

Use of a visual aid can improve accuracy of EBL after delivery. One study provided a pocket card to L&D providers with pictures of blood on common obstetric materials who then visited 6 simulated stations with known volumes of blood.[11] The visual aid did improve both objective and subjective estimation of blood loss. Interestingly, neither provider type nor years of experience correlated with accuracy either before or after using the intervention. Experienced anesthesiologists were no more accurate than obstetricians, nurses, or anesthesiology residents. Weighing sponges and other blood-containing materials will improve accuracy while keeping an ongoing estimation of blood loss. ACOG recommends quantitative methods of measuring obstetric blood loss such as graduated drapes or weighing, as these techniques provide a more accurate assessment of actual blood loss than visual estimation.[12] If there is concern for hemorrhage, bring a scale into the patient's room to weigh materials with blood on them and also keep a running total of all blood loss on a white board in her room where it can be viewed by all team members.

Uterotonic agents are the first-line treatment for postpartum hemorrhage. After ensuring adequate intravenous access, the anesthesia team should administer oxytocic medications. Anesthesiologists must know the dose, route, and major side effects of the oxytocic drugs that can be used (**Table 2**). Oxytocin is the mainstay of the uterotonic medications, but the optimal dose is unclear. Bolus doses $\geq$10 units

Obstetric Hemorrhage Checklist   EXAMPLE

Complete all steps in prior stages plus current stage regardless of stage in which the patient presents.

> Postpartum hemorrhage is defined as cumulative blood loss of greater than or equal to 1,000mL or blood loss accompanied by signs or symptoms of hypovolemia within 24 hours. However, blood loss >500mL in a vaginal delivery is abnormal, and should be investigated and managed as outlined in Stage 1.

RECOGNITION:

☐ Call for assistance (Obstetric Hemorrhage Team)

Designate: ☐ Team leader _____ ☐ Checklist reader/recorder ☐ Primary RN

Announce: ☐ Cumulative blood loss ☐ Vital signs _____ ☐ Determine stage

> **STAGE 1:** Blood loss >1000mL after delivery with normal vital signs and lab values. Vaginal delivery 500-999mL should be treated as in Stage 1.

INITIAL STEPS:

☐ Ensure 16G or 18G IV Access

☐ Increase IV fluid (crystalloid without oxytocin)

☐ Insert indwelling urinary catheter

☐ Fundal massage

MEDICATIONS:

☐ Ensure appropriate medications given patient history

☐ Increase oxytocin, additional uterotonics

BLOOD BANK:

☐ Confirm active type and screen and consider crossmatch of 2 units PRBCs

ACTION:

☐ Determine etiology and treat

☐ Prepare OR, if clinically indicated (optimize visualization/examination)

Oxytocin (Pitocin):
10-40 units per 500-1000mL solution

Methylergonovine (Methergine):
0.2 milligrams IM (may repeat);
Avoid with hypertension

15-methyl PGF₂α (Hemabate, Carboprost):
250 micrograms IM (may repeat in q15 minutes, maximum 8 doses); **Avoid with asthma; use with caution with hypertension**

Misoprostol (Cytotec):
800-1000 micrograms PR
600 micrograms PO or 800 micrograms SL

Tone (i.e., atony)
Trauma (i.e., laceration)
Tissue (i.e., retained products)
Thrombin (i.e., coagulation dysfunction)

> **STAGE 2:** Continued Bleeding (EBL up to 1500mL OR > 2 uterotonics) with normal vital signs and lab values

INITIAL STEPS:

☐ Mobilize additional help

☐ Place 2nd IV (16-18G)

☐ Draw STAT labs (CBC, Coags, Fibrinogen)

☐ Prepare OR

MEDICATIONS:

☐ Continue Stage 1 medications; consider TXA

BLOOD BANK:

☐ Obtain 2 units PRBCs (DO NOT wait for labs. Transfuse per clinical signs/symptoms)

☐ Thaw 2 units FFP

ACTION:

☐ For uterine atony --> consider uterine balloon or packing, possible surgical interventions

☐ Consider moving patient to OR

☐ Escalate therapy with goal of hemostasis

Tranexamic Acid (TXA)
1 gram IV over 10 min (add 1 gram vial to 100mL NS & give over 10 min; may be repeated once after 30 min)

Possible interventions:
• Bakri balloon
• Compression suture/B-Lynch suture
• Uterine artery ligation
• Hysterectomy

Huddle and move to Stage 3 if continued blood loss and/or abnormal VS

Safe Motherhood Initiative

ACOG
The American College of
Obstetricians and Gynecologists
District II

Revised June 2019

STAGE 3: Continued Bleeding (EBL > 1500mL OR > 2 RBCs given OR at risk for occult bleeding/ coagulopathy OR any patient with abnormal vital signs/labs/oliguria)

INITIAL STEPS:

☐ Mobilize additional help

☐ Move to OR

☐ Announce clinical status
(vital signs, cumulative blood loss, etiology)

☐ Outline and communicate plan

MEDICATIONS:

☐ Continue Stage 1 medications; consider TXA

BLOOD BANK:

☐ Initiate Massive Transfusion Protocol
(If clinical coagulopathy: add cryoprecipitate,
consult for additional agents)

ACTION:

☐ Achieve hemostasis, intervention based on etiology

☐ Escalate interventions

Oxytocin (Pitocin):
10-40 units per 500-1000mL solution

Methylergonovine (Methergine):
0.2 milligrams IM (may repeat);
Avoid with hypertension

15-methyl PGF$_2$α (Hemabate, Carboprost):
250 micrograms IM
(may repeat in q15 minutes, maximum 8 doses)
**Avoid with asthma;
use with caution with hypertension**

Misoprostol (Cytotec):
800-1000 micrograms PR
600 micrograms PO or 800 micrograms SL

Tranexamic Acid (TXA)
1 gram IV over 10 min (add 1 gram vial to
100mL NS & give over 10 min; may be repeated
once after 30 min)

Possible interventions:
• Bakri balloon
• Compression suture/B-Lynch suture
• Uterine artery ligation
• Hysterectomy

STAGE 4: Cardiovascular Collapse (massive hemorrhage, profound hypovolemic shock, or amniotic fluid embolism)

INITIAL STEP:

☐ Mobilize additional resources

MEDICATIONS:

☐ ACLS

BLOOD BANK:

☐ Simultaneous aggressive massive transfusion

ACTION:

☐ Immediate surgical intervention to ensure
hemostasis (hysterectomy)

Post-Hemorrhage Management

• Determine disposition of patient

• Debrief with the whole obstetric care team

• Debrief with patient and family

• Document

Revised June 2019

Safe Motherhood Initiative

Fig. 1. (continued).

Table 2
Oxytocic medications, dosing, and side effects

Medication	Dose and Route	Side Effects
Oxytocin[13]	10–80 units/L as an infusion	Intravenous (IV) bolus doses ≥10 units can cause vasodilation and hypotension, hyponatremia can occur when administered in hypotonic intravenous solutions.
Methylergonovine	0.2 mg intramuscular (IM)	As an ergot preparation can cause widespread vasoconstriction, increased pulmonary artery pressures, coronary artery vasospasm, systemic hypertension, nausea, and vomiting.
Prostaglandin $F_{2\alpha}$ (Carboprost)	0.25 mg IM	May cause bronchospasm, VQ mismatching with hypoxia, increased pulmonary artery pressures, nausea and diarrhea.
Misoprostol	400–800 μg buccal, rectal, vaginal or intrauterine	May cause acute hyperthermia in high doses.
Carbetocin[14]	100 μg IV	Minimal side effects but not available in the United States.

Data from Refs.[13,14]

can cause significant vasodilation and hypotension, especially in the presence of hypovolemia due to hemorrhage. In the United States, oxytocin is commonly administered as an infusion rather than a bolus dose. Studies comparing women having cesarean delivery without labor to those having cesarean delivery for the indication of labor dystocia have shown the ED_{90} of oxytocin is increased significantly after labor, presumably because of down-regulation of oxytocin receptors in the uterus. In an up-down sequential allocation dose-response study, the oxytocin ED_{90} infusion rate was 44.2 units/h in a laboring group requiring cesarean delivery compared with only 16.2 units/h in a nonlaboring group.[13] Significantly more women in the laboring group also required supplemental uterotonic agents (34% vs 8%). Supplemental agents may include methylergonovine (Methergine) and prostaglandins, with the choice often based on potential adverse effects (see **Table 2**). Carbetocin, an oxytocin analogue, is highly effective with minimal side effects, but is not available in the United States.[14]

Once the diagnosis of severe hemorrhage is made, the massive transfusion protocol will be ordered. This may include protocols that follow a 1 packed RBCs: 1 fresh frozen plasma (FFP): 1 platelet unit strategy, cell salvage, medications to manage coagulopathy such as tranexamic acid and recombinant Factor VIIa, point-of-care testing, and interventional radiology techniques[15] (**Table 3**). Peripartum resuscitation always includes maintenance of normal acid-base status and avoidance of hypothermia.

Fig. 1. An example of an obstetric hemorrhage checklist. (*From* The American College of Obstetricians and Gynecologists District II. Obstetric Hemorrhage Checklist. Available at: https://www.acog.org/-/media/project/acog/acogorg/files/forms/districts/smi-ob-hemorrhage-bundle-hemorrhage-checklist.pdf; with permission.)

Table 3
Management techniques for severe postpartum hemorrhage

Strategy	References
1:1:1 Transfusion protocols	16,17
Cell salvage	19–21
Fibrinogen levels, thromboelastography or rotational thromboelastometry, emergency hemostasis panel	22–25
Tranexamic acid	26,27
Recombinant Factor VIIa and other factor concentrates	28,29
Interventional radiology techniques	30–34
Resuscitative endovascular balloon occlusion (REBOA)	35,36
Obstetric techniques: uterine tamponade balloon, uterine compression sutures, vascular ligation and hysterectomy	1,10

Data from Refs.[7,15,18]

Despite the lack of randomized controlled trials in obstetric patients, many L&D units have adopted massive transfusion protocols similar to those used for military trauma cases and other types of traumatic injury.[16] These protocols focus on early administration of FFP and platelets with RBCs to achieve a ratio of 1:1:1 without waiting for laboratory tests of coagulation. There are limited data in obstetric patients, but a retrospective observational study of 142 women with postpartum hemorrhage found a higher FFP:RBC ratio was associated with a lower requirement for advanced interventional procedures such as embolization, B-Lynch suture, or hysterectomy.[17] A massive transfusion protocol for L&D based on established trauma protocols should expedite release of blood products in a 1:1:1 ratio, provide availability of a blood bank pathologist for consultation, describe standard responses for L&D team members that can be regularly practiced in simulations, and should mobilize resources for the laboratory to manage frequent assessment and rapid turnaround with the goal of improving patient safety and reducing utilization of blood products.[16,18]

Concern for amniotic fluid embolism syndrome (AFE) and for alloimmunization due to fetal RBC contamination has limited the use of RBC salvage during cesarean delivery. However, a comparison of maternal central venous blood with cell salvage blood after washing and with use of a leukocyte depletion filter showed no difference in particulate contaminants.[19] Over 400 case reports of cell salvage in parturients have been published with no cases of AFE attributed to infusion of cell salvaged blood. If banked blood cannot be cross-matched or the patient refuses transfusion, the use of cell salvage can be life-saving. In addition, cell salvage can be cost-effective and may decrease the incidence of infectious and non-infectious complications of banked blood transfusion.[19] Its use in obstetric hemorrhage is supported in practice guidelines from national bodies in the United States and Great Britain. However, one case report of a woman being resuscitated after presumed amniotic fluid embolism described acute hypotension and worsening of hemodynamics immediately after infusion of cell salvage blood was started.[20] It is possible that resuscitation during AFE syndrome is a unique exclusion to the use of cell salvage blood. Others have proposed that the leukocyte depletion filter used to minimize contamination by white cells and particulate components of amniotic fluid such as fetal squamous cells and phospholipid lamellar bodies may be a potential cause of hypotension.[21] Bradykinin production is a possible mechanism. While cell salvage may be useful if available, access to the equipment and a perfusionist may limit its use in acute or emergency situations on the L&D unit.

Laboratory studies are an integral part of resuscitation.[16] Fibrinogen levels, rotational thromboelastometry (ROTEM), and thromboelastography (TEG) may be particularly helpful in obstetric hemorrhage. Several studies have shown that a low fibrinogen level in the early phase of obstetric hemorrhage is an important predictor of severe postpartum hemorrhage.[22] Fibrinogen levels less than 2 g/L are independently associated with an increased risk of severe postpartum hemorrhage (OR 12.0, 95% CI 2.6–56.1). Placental abruption and AFE are particularly associated with critically low fibrinogen levels and early use of cryoprecipitate should be included for those diagnoses. ROTEM and TEG give a global picture of real-time clotting activity and can be used to guide component therapy. Reference ranges specific to the peripartum period have been established for ROTEM thromboelastometry.[23] A single-center study compared their outcomes before and after implementation of a ROTEM protocol used during postpartum hemorrhage.[24] The testing group received fewer packed RBCs and platelets, and their incidence of hysterectomy, intensive care unit (ICU) admission, and length of stay was less, making cost of hospitalization less. A criticism of standard coagulation tests has been their slow turnaround times. One institution described the multidisciplinary development of an emergency hemostasis panel composed of prothrombin time, fibrinogen concentration, platelet count and hemoglobin concentration.[25] By making adjustments in sample handling and calibration, the laboratory could provide results within 15 minutes. Both laboratory and point-of-care testing have value.

Pharmacologic therapy for severe obstetric hemorrhage may include antifibrinolytic agents such as tranexamic acid (TXA) and factor concentrates. Use these agents with caution in postpartum patients as they are at high risk of thrombotic events. Because fibrinolysis may be seen during severe peripartum hemorrhage, there has been interest in the use of TXA for prevention and treatment of postpartum hemorrhage. In 2017 the WOMAN (World Maternal Antifibrinolytic Randomized) Trial was published.[26] In a global randomized trial, 20,000 women received 1 g TXA or placebo at the time postpartum hemorrhage was diagnosed. In the group receiving TXA, there was no increase in adverse events including thrombotic complications, and mortality due to bleeding was reduced by 19% overall and by 31% if given within 3 hours of delivery. TXA appears to be a safe, effective and inexpensive option in the management of postpartum hemorrhage, but its prophylactic use is not routinely recommended since it crosses the placenta and newborn effects are unknown. It can also cause seizures and death if accidently administered intrathecally, for example, if ampules are switched during placement of spinal anesthesia. Most countries in the WOMAN trial were low resource countries, for example, 7% of women were not even transfused before death and interventions such as the Bakri balloon or B-Lynch suture were uncommon, so the relevance of the results in a high resource country such as the United States is unclear. However, a decision tree analysis using US data and 3 groups: no TXA, TXA administered at any time after delivery, and TXA given within 3 hours of delivery or postpartum hemorrhage found that giving TXA at any point would prevent 9 maternal deaths per year and $11.3 million in expense.[27] Administration within 3 hours of hemorrhage tripled savings and improved outcomes even further. TXA should be part of the protocol for managing postpartum hemorrhage.

Nonrandomized case series using recombinant Factor VIIa (rFVIIa; NovoSeven) for postpartum hemorrhage were encouraging, but a randomized controlled trial of 84 women unresponsive to uterotonics found that although administration of rFVIIa reduced the need for secondary therapies such as transfusion, hysterectomy or interventional radiology procedures by 41% (from 93% to 52%), 1 in 20 had thrombotic complications.[28] They concluded it was an expensive therapy that failed almost half the time and resulted in thrombotic complications in 5%. Its use in AFE syndrome has also been challenged. A case series of 44 reports of AFE compared those who received rFVIIa with those who did not and found the risk of death or permanent disability was doubled when rFVIIa was given.[29] Although there are methodologic problems with this type of study, the results are concerning. During AFE, high circulating tissue factor concentrations can combine with rFVIIa to form intravascular clots. Because post-procedure thromboembolism is a major concern, thromboprophylaxis is recommended once bleeding risk is low. If used, rFVIIa is most effective when the patient is normothermic, has a normal acid-base status and ionized calcium level, and platelets and clotting factors have been replaced. Other factor concentrates have not been studied in obstetric patients although there is no contraindication to their use.

Consultation with an interventional radiologist provides another therapeutic option for real or potential uncontrolled hemorrhage. Balloon or embolization catheters can be placed into the iliac vessels by a femoral route either preoperatively[30,31] or when life-threatening hemorrhage has not responded to other treatments. Occlusion or embolization of the iliac, hypogastric or uterine vessels can treat hemorrhage after vaginal or cesarean deliveries when other measures have not been successful. Fertility is preserved and success rates as high as 80% to 90% have been reported in some series.[32] The technique seems to be less effective in the presence of coagulopathy or during acute massive hemorrhage, and should not replace ongoing resuscitation and transfusion or delay proceeding with hysterectomy when necessary. The "ideal" candidate for embolization would be hemodynamically stable, appear to have persistent slow bleeding, and have failed less invasive therapy. Prophylactic placement of catheters can also be considered as part of a multi-modal treatment plan before cesarean delivery when placenta accreta or percreta has been diagnosed antepartum or when the patient refuses blood products for religious or other reasons.[30,31,33] Serious complications are rare but can occur with these techniques, including leg ischemia, tissue necrosis, pseudoaneurysms, and even paraplegia.[34]

Obstetric management of postpartum hemorrhage will include additional therapies such as uterine massage, tamponade techniques such as a Bakri balloon, uterine compression sutures such as the B-Lynch technique, bilateral uterine artery ligation with O'Leary sutures, and ultimately hysterectomy.[1] The Resuscitative Endovascular Balloon Occlusion of the Aorta (REBOA) device has been used in traumatic hemorrhagic shock and has been described for obstetric patients.[35] The balloon catheter is inserted by a trauma surgeon into the femoral artery and threaded into the aorta, so that when inflated it acts as an internal aortic cross-clamp. For obstetric hemorrhage the balloon is deployed in Zone 3 below the renal arteries. Deployment should be for less than 60 minutes to prevent ischemia, end organ damage, and reperfusion injury.[36] In an extreme situation when arterial bleeding has been controlled and persistent bleeding is deemed due to coagulopathy refractory to blood product replacement, consider damage-control surgery with abdomino-pelvic packing followed by medical stabilization in the ICU.[37]

Unique Obstetric Conditions that Lead to Severe Peripartum Hemorrhage

Obstetric hemorrhage can occur antepartum or postpartum; when antepartum, both mother and fetus are at risk of harm. The following conditions are unique to the parturient and contribute to peripartum hemorrhage. They are discussed in terms of their etiology and risk factors, method of diagnosis, obstetric management, and anesthetic considerations.

Antepartum:	Abnormal placentation: previa and vasa previa/accreta/increta/percreta Placental abruption Uterine rupture Ruptured ectopic pregnancy
Postpartum:	Uterine atony Uterine inversion AFE

ANTEPARTUM MATERNAL HEMORRHAGE
Abnormal Placentation: Placenta Previa/Vasa Previa/Accreta/Increta/Percreta

Definitions and risk factors
A placenta previa exists when all or part of the placenta lies over the cervical os in front of the fetal presenting part. Vasa previa is a condition in which unprotected fetal blood vessels run through the membranes over the cervix and are at high risk of rupture during labor, leading to fetal death.[38] Placenta accreta is an abnormally adherent placenta in which chorionic villi attach to the myometrium. It accounts for 78% of accreta spectrum cases. There is a spectrum of variants of placenta accreta, depending on depth of invasion. A placenta increta (17% of cases) has grown into the myometrium, whereas a placenta percreta (5% of cases) has grown through the myometrium and uterine serosa with or without invasion into other pelvic structures such as bladder, bowel or vasculature.[39]

Risk factors for abnormal placentation include uterine scarring from prior cesarean delivery or myomectomy, uterine fibroids, a history of postpartum hemorrhage, and multiparity. The greatest risk for placenta accreta is placenta previa in the presence of prior cesarean delivery. The risk is highly related to the number of previous uterine scars (usually cesarean sections) in the presence of a placenta previa.[40] (Table 4) As the number of prior cesarean deliveries goes up, a woman with a placenta previa faces increasing maternal morbidity from coagulopathy, hysterectomy, thromboembolism and pulmonary edema.[41] In the presence of placenta previa, composite maternal morbidity is 15% if she has never had a cesarean delivery, 23% with one prior cesarean, 59% with 2 prior cesareans, and 83% with 3 or more cesarean deliveries. Perinatal morbidity is not affected, although antepartum diagnosis of abnormal placentation may lead to a planned preterm delivery.

Table 4
Association between the presence of placenta previa, prior cesarean deliveries, and risk of placenta accreta spectrum with resultant maternal morbidity

Number of Prior Cesarean Deliveries	Risk of Placenta Accreta,[40] %	Composite Maternal Morbidity,[41] %
0	3	15
1	11	23
2	40	59
≥3	61	83

Data from Refs.[39–42]

Diagnosis

Placenta previa usually presents as painless vaginal bleeding in the third trimester. The first episode of bleeding is often mild (a "sentinel" bleed), but subsequent bleeds may be catastrophic. A digital cervical examination should never be performed on a patient with vaginal bleeding before an ultrasound to locate the position of the placenta. The presence of placenta previa in the setting of prior cesarean delivery should prompt further workup for placenta accreta and preparation for potentially massive hemorrhage at the time of delivery.

Placenta accreta may not be diagnosed until after delivery when the placenta does not separate normally at vaginal or cesarean delivery, but more commonly there are characteristic antepartum ultrasound findings such as loss of the normal hypoechoic retroplacental zone or vascular lacunae (irregular vascular spaces) within the placenta.[42] However one report found that when ultrasounds from patients with clinically diagnosed placenta accreta were given to blinded but experienced clinicians, there was a false negative rate of 18.3%. This implies that almost 1 in 5 cases may be missed based on their antepartum ultrasound findings. MRI may be helpful if ultrasound is inconclusive or if placenta percreta is suspected.[42]

Obstetric management

Once placenta previa is diagnosed by ultrasound, an elective cesarean delivery will be scheduled. If the fetus is immature, the patient may be managed expectantly in the hospital until the fetus has received steroids for lung maturity or until further bleeding occurs. Active labor or persistent bleeding will require an urgent trip to the operating room.

The management of placenta accreta or percreta requires early recognition by the obstetrician and a decision to proceed with cesarean hysterectomy.[42] Leaving the placenta in situ without hysterectomy is a less commonly used approach. If extensive adherence to pelvic sidewalls or bladder is documented at the time of delivery, if the patient strongly desires future fertility, or if transfusion is not an option, the surgeon may opt to leave the placenta in situ to involute with or without use of methotrexate.[43] This technique has unpredictable results and requires close follow-up because of the risk of infection or further bleeding, but may be life-saving if the patient refuses blood transfusion or adequate blood products are not available.[30,31] Cesarean hysterectomy with the placenta left in situ remains the treatment of choice.[42] Management of placenta percreta usually requires the presence of additional surgical specialties to manage vascular involvement or dissection of the bowel or bladder. If interventional radiology techniques are being considered, delivery in a hybrid operating suite that combines a general surgical suite and interventional radiology capability is preferable so the patient does not have to be moved after placement of catheters.[44]

Anesthetic considerations

The anesthetic management of placenta previa includes:

- Evaluation of the airway in case emergency general anesthesia is required,
- Large-bore intravenous (IV) access (preferably 2 18- or 16-gauge catheters),
- Having a Level 1 or equivalent fluid warmer available, and
- Verifying that cross-matched blood is available in the Blood Bank.

There is no evidence that neuraxial anesthesia should be avoided during cesarean delivery for placenta previa. Two retrospective reviews of 514 and 350 cases of placenta previa found neuraxial anesthesia was associated with reduced blood loss and reduced need for transfusion compared with general anesthesia.[45,46] Conversion from neuraxial to general anesthesia was only required for inadequate duration of 2 spinal anesthetics during hysterectomy for placenta accreta. Vasoactive drugs should be immediately available, as well as skilled assistance and ultrasound to place invasive monitoring if needed.

The most important aspect of anesthetic management of placenta accreta or percreta is awareness of a patient's risk factors and communication with the obstetrics team, initially in the form of a multidisciplinary care conference that involves nursing and other surgical consultants. A checklist can be used to assure all aspects of delivery care including site, resources, personnel and surgical approach have been addressed.[42,47] Small hospitals or institutions with insufficient blood bank supply or inadequate availability of subspecialty and support personnel should consider patient transfer to a Level III or Level IV maternal care center.[48]

The risk of major blood loss associated with cesarean hysterectomy in these cases necessitates large-bore IV access, arterial line placement, a pressure/warming system for administering fluids and blood products, rapid availability of cross-matched blood with the ability to institute a massive transfusion protocol, and additional personnel to assist with resuscitation and central line placement if needed.[16,49] Hysterectomy and massive transfusion will usually require general endotracheal anesthesia. If the woman is highly motivated to be awake to see her newborn, the case can be started using a combined spinal-epidural technique with general anesthesia induced after delivery, and the epidural used for postoperative pain management.

Placental Abruption

Risk factors
Known risk factors for placental abruption include hypertension, advanced age and parity, smoking, cocaine use, abdominal trauma, premature rupture of membranes, and history of previous abruption.

Diagnosis
As the placenta separates from the decidua, bleeding occurs from the exposed vessels, and fetal distress develops because there is less area for maternal-fetal gas exchange. Although the classic presentation is vaginal bleeding with uterine tenderness, hypertonicity and fetal distress, the presentation can be extremely variable. The abruption may or may not be visible on ultrasound and vaginal bleeding may not occur if the clot is retroplacental.

Obstetric management
Initial management includes evaluation of fetal well-being with heart rate monitoring and biophysical profile, placement of large-bore intravenous lines, type-and-crossmatch of blood products, and obtaining maternal hematocrit and coagulation studies.[50] The maternal risks of abruption are significant hemorrhage and coagulopathy while fetal risks include hypoxia and prematurity. Although delivery of the fetus is the definitive treatment, the route of delivery and timing depends on the condition of the mother and fetus. Severe fetal distress or maternal hemodynamic instability necessitates urgent cesarean delivery. However, if the fetus and mother are stable and the cervical examination is favorable, induction of labor and vaginal delivery may be attempted.

Anesthetic considerations
There is no contraindication to regional anesthesia for labor or cesarean delivery if maternal volume status and coagulation studies including fibrinogen are normal. However, if the mother is hemodynamically unstable or coagulopathic and general

anesthesia is planned, etomidate or ketamine may be preferable to propofol for induction to maintain hemodynamic stability. Aggressive volume replacement may be necessary, and invasive monitoring with an arterial line for blood draws may be helpful. A urinary catheter will help to assess volume status. Uterine atony is common after delivery of the placenta, and additional oxytocic drugs such as methylergonovine and prostaglandins should be available.

Uterine Rupture

Risk factors
Conditions associated with uterine rupture include prior uterine surgery, abdominal trauma, direct uterine trauma following forceps delivery or curettage, grand multiparity, and fetal macrosomia or malposition. The risk of uterine rupture in pregnancy after a low transverse uterine incision is 0.5% to 0.9%. Concern for uterine rupture during a trial of labor after cesarean delivery has led to more stringent practice guidelines including the immediate availability of all personnel necessary to perform emergency cesarean delivery.[51] Several factors increase the likelihood of a *failed* trial of labor, which in turn is associated with increased maternal and perinatal morbidity when compared with a successful trial of labor (ie, vaginal birth after cesarean [VBAC]) or with elective repeat cesarean delivery. An individual patient's chance of a successful VBAC can be calculated using the on-line Maternal-Fetal Medicine Units Network Vaginal Birth After Cesarean calculator (https://mfmunetwork.bsc.gwu.edu/PublicBSC/MFMU/VGBirthCalc/vagbirth.html).

Diagnosis
In the appropriate clinical setting, uterine rupture should be suspected when there is fetal distress, shoulder pain (due to blood in the abdomen irritating the diaphragm), abdominal pain between contractions and unrelieved by epidural analgesia, loss of fetal station or change in fetal presenting part, sudden maternal hemodynamic instability, cessation of uterine contractions on an intrauterine pressure catheter, or rarely vaginal bleeding. Pain is not a sensitive indicator and fetal distress is the most common presenting sign.

Obstetric management
Dehiscence of a prior uterine scar is far more common than catastrophic uterine rupture.[52,53] Suspected dehiscence or rupture should prompt immediate delivery. Depending on the condition of the uterus, the obstetrician may be able to repair the dehiscence or rupture, but hysterectomy is sometimes required.

Anesthetic considerations
Anesthetic involvement often begins during an emergency cesarean delivery for fetal distress, with the uterine rupture discovered intraoperatively. General anesthesia may be necessary if (1) the case is emergent and a functioning epidural catheter is not in place for labor analgesia, (2) if there is hemodynamic instability due to blood loss, or (3) if hysterectomy is required.

Rupture of an Ectopic Pregnancy

Risk factors
Hemorrhage from ruptured ectopic pregnancy is the leading cause of pregnancy-related maternal death in the first trimester. The most common implantation site outside the uterus is the fallopian tube. The major risk factors for ectopic pregnancy are previous conservative treatment for ectopic pregnancy (15% recurrence), tubal

pathology from infection or surgery, and in utero diethylstilbestrol (DES) exposure, but many patients have no documented risk factors.

Diagnosis
Patients will present with abdominal or pelvic pain, and hemorrhagic shock may develop if rupture has occurred. If the ectopic pregnancy is intact, a serum human chorionic gonadotropin and a transvaginal ultrasound examination will determine whether the patient is pregnant and whether the pregnancy is intrauterine. Depending on gestational age, an adnexal mass may be seen.[54]

Obstetric/gynecologic management
Once the diagnosis of a ruptured ectopic pregnancy is made, the patient will be taken to the operating room for removal of the affected fallopian tube or dissection of the ectopic pregnancy with preservation of the tube. Laparoscopy is the preferred surgical approach, but if there is extensive bleeding or poor visualization of the pelvis, laparotomy should be performed.[54]

Anesthetic management
General endotracheal anesthesia will be required for this emergent laparoscopic or open abdominal procedure. If she is hemodynamically unstable, obtain large-bore intravenous access, ensure that cross-matched blood is available, use vasopressor support, have access to invasive monitors if needed, and maintain normothermia. Postoperative nausea and vomiting (PONV) prophylaxis should also be given for this patient with many risk factors for PONV.

POSTPARTUM MATERNAL HEMORRHAGE
Uterine Atony

Risk factors
Uterine contraction is the primary mechanism controlling blood loss at delivery, and thus uterine atony is the most common cause of postpartum hemorrhage, accounting for 75% to 80% of cases.[55] Conditions associated with atony include the following:

Multiple gestation	Chorioamnionitis
Macrosomia	Precipitous labor
Polyhydramnios	Prolonged labor
High parity (>5)	Augmented labor (exposure to oxytocin)
Prior postpartum hemorrhage	Volatile anesthetics (>0.5 minimum alveolar concentration)
Maternal age < 20 or > 40	Tocolytic use (eg, nifedipine, magnesium)
Obesity	Retained placenta

However, more than 60% of cases have no recognized risk factors.

Diagnosis
Uterine atony is diagnosed after vaginal or cesarean delivery by manual examination of the uterine fundus that demonstrates lack of firmness and muscle tone.

Obstetric management
In addition to infusion of oxytocin, the obstetrician will perform bimanual compression of the uterus, uterine massage, and evaluation for retained placenta. Retained placenta can be seen on ultrasound examination and may be removed by a manual sweep or by curettage. Additional oxytocic medications will be administered (see **Table 2**). If hemorrhage continues, other strategies for obstetric management may

include placement of an intrauterine balloon catheter for tamponade of the uterus and use of compression sutures.[1]

Anesthetic considerations
The patient should be evaluated for hemodynamic stability and need for analgesia. The necessary obstetric maneuvers can be extremely painful, especially for a patient who has had an unmedicated birth. Oxygen should be administered and monitors placed for blood pressure and heart rate. If blood loss is ongoing, additional intravenous access should be obtained for volume replacement. Blood samples should be sent for baseline hematocrit and coagulation studies including fibrinogen. If the patient does not have a regional anesthetic in place and requires short-term analgesia for obstetric maneuvers, inhaled nitrous oxide or intravenous fentanyl or ketamine may be given. If the patient is still in a labor room setting, consider moving to the operating room so that general anesthesia can be induced if necessary, patient position and lighting can be optimized for the obstetrician, and aggressive resuscitation can be more easily performed. Consider implementing the massive transfusion protocol with ongoing blood loss.[15]

Uterine Inversion

Etiology
Uterine inversion is an uncommon but life-threatening problem often associated with fundal pressure during delivery or excessive traction on the umbilical cord, especially if placenta accreta is present and the placenta does not easily separate. The uterine fundus collapses into the endometrial cavity, turning the uterus partially or completely inside out.

Diagnosis
The diagnosis is usually obvious. There will be massive hemorrhage due to atony, vasovagal shock due to traction on the uterosacral ligaments, and a mass in the vagina or outside the perineum. Maternal hypotension and cardiovascular collapse develop rapidly.

Obstetric management
Rapid replacement of the uterus is required by pushing a hand against the everted fundus up into the uterine cavity, followed by oxytocic drugs and uterine massage to maintain uterine tone.

Anesthetic considerations
Uterine relaxation is often necessary before the uterus can be replaced, and intense analgesia for the procedure is also required.[1,56] Rapid induction of general anesthesia with intubation and volatile anesthetics could accomplish both of these objectives. However, since most deliveries occur outside the operating room, general anesthesia is rarely practical. If the patient does not have an epidural in place for delivery and is uncomfortable or unable to cooperate, intravenous ketamine (25–50 mg) for analgesia plus a uterine relaxant such as nitroglycerin (100–500 µg IV or 400 µg sublingual) or terbutaline (250 µg subcutaneously or IV) can be used in the labor room setting. Volume resuscitation must occur simultaneously, and additional assistance is key. Blood loss can be massive, so large-bore IV access and transfusion is often necessary.

Nitroglycerin has a fast onset and short duration when used in an intravenous bolus or sublingual dose for tocolysis.[57] Short duration is an important benefit since uterine atony after replacement is common, and administration of oxytocics should begin immediately. The mechanism of action of nitroglycerin in causing uterine relaxation is unknown, although nitric oxide's effects on smooth muscle may play a role. A wide range of bolus doses has been described, from 50 to 1500 mcg intravenously. Since it is a vasodilator, when used in the presence of hypovolemia it should be accompanied by a pressor such as phenylephrine and volume resuscitation as appropriate.

Amniotic Fluid Embolism

Etiology

AFE is a rare event unique to obstetrics with mortality rates of 20% to 60% and high morbidity; 61% of survivors have clinically significant neurologic consequences.[58] It is completely unpredictable and the etiology is unknown, but it is not actually an embolism and is not caused by amniotic fluid. The pathophysiology appears to involve an abnormal maternal response (sometimes described as anaphylactoid) to fetal tissue exposure associated with breaches of the maternal-fetal physiologic barrier in the peripartum period. This reaction and its subsequent injury seem to involve activation of proinflammatory mediators similar to that seen with the classic systemic inflammatory response syndrome.[59] There is a biphasic pattern of sudden cardiovascular collapse in the immediate peripartum period, initially from vasospasm of the pulmonary vasculature and right heart failure, followed by left heart compression by the dilated right ventricle, decreased filling pressure, heart failure and elevated pulmonary artery pressures.[58]

Diagnosis

The diagnosis of AFE is one of exclusion, but is based on the classic triad of hemodynamic and respiratory compromise accompanied by disseminated intravascular coagulopathy. The differential may include pulmonary embolism, venous air embolism, anaphylaxis, high cephalad spread of neuraxial anesthesia, peripartum cardiomyopathy, intrapartum myocardial infarction, or eclampsia.[58]

Obstetric management

The obstetrician should evaluate for other sources of bleeding such as uterine lacerations or retained placenta. While active resuscitation is ongoing, if uterine atony cannot be managed with uterotonics and other techniques such as tamponade suturing, hysterectomy should be done expeditiously to prevent a delay in definitive bleeding control.[58]

Anesthetic considerations

Additional assistance is crucial. In 87% of cases cardiac arrest will occur and high-quality cardiopulmonary resuscitation with chest compressions should begin.[60] If the patient is still pregnant at the time of arrest, preparations should be made immediately for cesarean delivery within 5 minutes, without moving the patient. Transesophageal echocardiography can be very helpful to manage pulmonary hypertension and cardiac failure, guiding the administration of pressors and inotropes as well as pulmonary vasodilators. Institute the massive transfusion protocol and manage coagulopathy with blood products as indicated by laboratory studies and point-of-care testing.[16] Consider preparing for extracorporeal membrane oxygenation (ECMO).[61] A series of 17 cases of AFE using ECMO as part of the resuscitation had a maternal survival of 85% and length of ICU stay from 7 to 59 days.

SUMMARY

All providers on L&D should be prepared to treat obstetric hemorrhage. A number of multidisciplinary groups including the National Partnership for Maternal Safety have created consensus bundles for treating obstetric hemorrhage that address "best practices" for this scenario.[7,10,62,63] These bundles stress recognizing risk factors for severe hemorrhage, preparing the L&D unit for patients at high risk, recognition and rapid response when hemorrhage does occur, and open reporting and tracking of hemorrhage events so contributing systems issues can be identified and corrected. Such initiatives are crucial as we continue working to reduce hemorrhage-related maternal morbidity and mortality.

REFERENCES

1. Postpartum hemorrhage. Practice Bulletin No. 183. American College of Obstetricians and Gynecologists. Obstet Gynecol 2017;130:e168–86 (reaffirmed 2019).
2. Peterson EE, Davis NL, Goodman D, et al. Pregnancy-related deaths, United States, 2011-2015 and strategies for prevention. MMWR Morb Mortal Wkly Rep 2019;68:423–9.
3. Say L, Chou D, Gemmill A, et al. Global causes of maternal death: a WHO systematic analysis. Lancet Glob Health 2014;2(6):e323–33.
4. Grobman WA, Bailit JL, Rice MM, et al. Frequency of and factors associated with severe maternal morbidity. Obstet Gynecol 2014;123:804–10.
5. Dutton RP, Lee LA, Stephens LS, et al. Massive hemorrhage: a report from the anesthesia closed claims project. Anesthesiology 2014;121:450–8.
6. Main EK, McCain CL, Morton CH, et al. Pregnancy-related mortality in California. Causes, characteristics, and improvement opportunities. Obstet Gynecol 2015; 125:938–47.
7. Main EK, Goffman D, Scavone BM, et al. National partnership for maternal safety: consensus bundle on obstetric hemorrhage. Anesth Analg 2015;121:143–8.
8. Kramer MS, Berg C, Abenhaim H, et al. Incidence, risk factors, and temporal trends in severe postpartum hemorrhage. Am J Obstet Gynecol 2013;209: 449.e1-7.
9. Mhyre JM, Shilkrut A, Kuklina EV, et al. Massive blood transfusion during hospitalization for delivery in New York State, 1998-2007. Obstet Gynecol 2013;122: 1288–94.
10. Available at: https://www.acog.org/community/districts-and-sections/district-ii/programs-and-resources/safe-motherhood-initiative/obstetric-hemorrhage. Accessed April 1, 2020.
11. Zuckerwise LC, Pettker CM, Illuzzi J, et al. Use of a novel visual aid to improve estimation of obstetric blood loss. Obstet Gynecol 2014;123:982–6.
12. Quantitative blood loss in obstetric hemorrhage. ACOG Committee Opinion No. 794. American College of Obstetricians and Gynecologists. Obstet Gynecol 2019;134:e150–6.
13. Lavoie A, McCarthy RJ, Wong CA. The ED_{90} of prophylactic oxytocin infusion after delivery of the placenta during cesarean delivery in laboring compared with nonlaboring women: an up-down sequential allocation dose-response study. Anesth Analg 2015;121:159–64.
14. Su LL, Chong YS, Samuel M. Carbetocin for preventing postpartum haemorrhage. Cochrane Database Syst Rev 2012;(4):CD005457.
15. Pacheco LD, Saade GR, Costantine MM, et al. An update on the use of massive transfusion protocols in obstetrics. Am J Obstet Gynecol 2016;214:340–4.
16. Pavord S, Maybury H. How I treat postpartum hemorrhage. Blood 2015;125: 2759–70.

17. Pasquier P, Gayat E, Rackelboom T, et al. An observational study of the fresh frozen plasma: red blood cell ratio in postpartum hemorrhage. Anesth Analg 2013;116:155–61.
18. Shields LE, Weisner S, Fulton J, et al. Comprehensive maternal hemorrhage protocols reduce the use of blood products and improve patient safety. Am J Obstet Gynecol 2015;212:272–80.
19. Goucher H, Wong CA, Patel SK, et al. Cell salvage in obstetrics. Anesth Analg 2015;121:465–8.
20. Rogers WK, Wernimont SA, Kumar GC, et al. Acute hypotension associated with intraoperative cell salvage using a leukocyte depletion filter during management of obstetric hemorrhage due to amniotic fluid embolism. Anesth Analg 2013;117: 449–52.
21. Sreelakshmi TR, Eldridge J. Acute hypotension associated with leucocyte depletion filters during cell salvaged blood transfusion. Anaesthesia 2010;65:742–4.
22. Butwick AJ. Postpartum hemorrhage and low fibrinogen levels: the past, present and future. Int J Obstet Anesth 2013;22:87–91.
23. deLange NM, van Rheenen-Flach LE, Lance MD, et al. Peri-partum reference ranges for ROTEM® thromboelastometry. Br J Anaesth 2014;112:852–9.
24. Snegovskikh D, Souza D, Walton Z, et al. Point-of-care viscoelastic testing improves the outcome of pregnancies complicated by severe postpartum hemorrhage. J Clin Anesth 2018;44:50–6.
25. Chandler WL. Emergency assessment of hemostasis in the bleeding patient. Int J Lab Hematol 2013;35:339–43.
26. WOMAN Trial Collaborators. Effect of early tranexamic acid administration on mortality, hysterectomy, and other morbidities in women with post-partum haemorrhage (WOMAN): an international, randomised, double-blind, placebo-controlled trial. Lancet 2017;389:2105–16.
27. Sudhof LS, Shainker SA, Einerson BD. Tranexamic acid in the routine treatment of postpartum hemorrhage in the United States: a cost-effectiveness analysis. Am J Obstet Gynecol 2019;221:275.e1-12.
28. Lavigne-Lassalde G, Aya AG, Mercier FJ, et al. Recombinant human FVIIa for reducing the need for invasive second-line therapies in severe refractory postpartum hemorrhage: a multicenter, randomized, open controlled trial. J Thromb Haemost 2015;13:520–9.
29. Leighton BL, Wall MH, Lockhart EM, et al. Use of recombinant factor VIIa in patients with amniotic fluid embolism. Anesthesiology 2011;115:1201–8.
30. Weinstein A, Chandra P, Schiavello H, et al. Conservative management of placenta previa percreta in a Jehovah's Witness. Obstet Gynecol 2005;105: 1247–50.
31. Mauritz AA, Dominguez JE, Guinn NR, et al. Blood conservation strategies in a blood-refusal parturient with placenta previa and placenta percreta. A A Case Rep 2016;6:111–3.
32. Ruiz Labarta FJ, Pintado Recarte MP, Alvarez Luque A, et al. Outcomes of pelvic arterial embolization in the management of postpartum haemorrhage: a case series study and systematic review. Eur J Obstet Gynecol Reprod Biol 2016;206: 12–21.
33. Mason CL, Tran CK. Caring for the Jehovah's Witness parturient. Anesth Analg 2015;121:1564–9.
34. Al-Thunyan A, Al-Meshal O, Al-Hussainan H, et al. Buttock necrosis and paraplegia after bilateral internal iliac artery embolization for postpartum hemorrhage. Obstet Gynecol 2012;120:468–70.

35. Sridhar S, Gumbert SD, Stephens C, et al. Resuscitative endovascular balloon occlusion of the aorta: principles, initial clinical experience, and considerations for the anesthesiologist. Anesth Analg 2017;125:884–90.
36. Joseph B, Zeeshan M, Sakran JV, et al. Nationwide analysis of resuscitative endovascular balloon occlusion of the aorta in civilian trauma. JAMA Surg 2019; 154:500–8.
37. Pacheco LD, Lozada MJ, Saade GR, et al. Damage-control surgery for obstetric hemorrhage. Obstet Gynecol 2018;132:423–7.
38. Matsuzaki S, Kimura T. Vasa previa. N Engl J Med 2019;380:274.
39. Silver RM, Ware Branch D. Placenta accreta spectrum. N Engl J Med 2018;378: 1529–36.
40. Silver RM, Landon MB, Rouse DJ, et al. Maternal morbidity associated with multiple repeat cesarean deliveries. Obstet Gynecol 2006;107:1226–32.
41. Grobman WA, Gersnoviez R, Landon MB, et al. Pregnancy outcomes for women with placenta previa in relation to the number of prior cesarean deliveries. Obstet Gynecol 2007;110:1249–55.
42. Placenta accreta spectrum. Obstetric Care Consensus No. 7. American College of Obstetricians and Gynecologists. Obstet Gynecol 2018;132:e259–75.
43. Pather S, Strockyj S, Richards A, et al. Maternal outcome after conservative management of placenta percreta at caesarean section: a report of three cases and a review of the literature. Aust N Z J Obstet Gynaecol 2014;54:84–7.
44. Clark A, Farber MK, Sviggum H, et al. Cesarean delivery in the hybrid operating suite: a promising new location for high-risk obstetric procedures. Anesth Analg 2013;117:1187–9.
45. Frederiksen MC, Glassenberg R, Stika CS. Placenta previa: a 22-year analysis. Am J Obstet Gynecol 1999;180:1432–7.
46. Parekh N, Husaini WU, Russell IF. Caesarean section for placenta praevia: a retrospective study of anaesthetic management. Br J Anaesth 2000;84:725–30.
47. Collins SL, Alemdar B, van Beekhuizen HJ, et al. Evidence-based guidelines for the management of abnormally invasive placenta: recommendations from the International Society for Abnormally Invasive Placenta. Am J Obstet Gynecol 2019; 220:511–26.
48. Levels of maternal care. Obstetric Care Consensus No. 9. American College of Obstetricians and Gynecologists. Obstet Gynecol 2019;134:e41–55.
49. Konishi Y, Yamamoto S, Sugiki K, et al. A novel and multidisciplinary strategy for cesarean delivery with placenta percreta: intraoperative embolization in a hybrid suite. A A Case Rep 2016;7:135–8.
50. Cunningham FG, Nelson DB. Disseminated intravascular coagulation syndromes in obstetrics. Obstet Gynecol 2015;126:999–1011.
51. American College of Obstetricians and Gynecologists. ACOG Practice Bulletin No. 205: Vaginal birth after cesarean delivery. Obstet Gynecol 2019;133: e110–27.
52. Eller AG, Fisher B. Diagnosis of uterine rupture on CT. N Engl J Med 2009; 360:170.
53. Bouet PE, Herondelle C. Uterine rupture with protruded legs in a large amniocele. N Engl J Med 2016;375:e51.
54. American College of Obstetricians and Gynecologists. Practice Bulletin No. 193: tubal ectopic pregnancy. Obstet Gynecol 2018;131:e91–103.
55. Bateman BT, Berman MF, Riley LE, et al. The epidemiology of postpartum hemorrhage in a large, nationwide sample of deliveries. Anesth Analg 2010;110: 1368–73.

56. Beringer RM, Patteril M. Puerperal uterine inversion and shock. Br J Anaesth 2004;92:439–41.
57. Wong RW, Greenfield MLVH, Polley LS. Nitroglycerin for uterine inversion in the absence of placental fragments. Anesth Analg 2006;103:511–2.
58. Bernstein SN, Cudemus-Deseda GA, Ortiz VE, et al. Case 33-2019: a 35-year old woman with cardiopulmonary arrest during cesarean section. N Engl J Med 2019; 381:1664–73.
59. Clark SL. Amniotic fluid embolism. Obstet Gynecol 2014;123:337–48.
60. Pacheco LD, Clark SL, Klassen M, et al. Amniotic fluid embolism: principles of early clinical management. Am J Obstet Gynecol 2020;222:48–52.
61. Viau-Lapointe J, Filewod N. Extracorporeal therapies for amniotic fluid embolism. Obstet Gynecol 2019;134:989.
62. Munoz M, Stensballe J, Ducloy-Bouthors AS, et al. Patient blood management in obstetrics: prevention and treatment of postpartum haemorrhage. A NATA consensus statement. Blood Transfus 2019;17:112–36.
63. Available at: https://www.cmqcc.org/resources-tool-kits/toolkits/ob-hemorrhage-toolkit. Accessed April 9, 2020.

Intraoperative Cardiac Arrest

Benjamin T. Houseman, MD, PhD[a], Joshua A. Bloomstone, MD, MSc[b,c,d],
Gerald Maccioli, MD, MBA[e],*

KEYWORDS

- Perioperative cardiac arrest • Crisis management • Resuscitation • Dynamic indices
- Local anesthetic systemic toxicity • Malignant hyperthermia • Anaphylaxis

KEY POINTS

- Unlike cardiac arrest in other settings, perioperative cardiac arrest (POCA) is often anticipated and managed by practitioners with detailed knowledge of the patient's medical and procedural history.
- Preventing POCA requires that anesthesiologists rapidly recognize early signs of crisis and initiate appropriate escalation of care.
- When POCA occurs, it frequently involves factors that are not explicitly addressed in conventional algorithms, such as advanced cardiac life support.
- Formulation of an appropriate diagnosis and rapid application of interventions aimed at treating the underlying cause of cardiac arrest are essential for optimizing outcomes.

INTRODUCTION

Cardiac arrest in the operating room (OR) and in the immediate postoperative period is a potentially catastrophic event that is almost always witnessed and is frequently anticipated.[1,2] Unlike cardiac arrest that occurs in nonhospital settings, staff members know the medical and surgical history of patients who suffer arrest in the perioperative period, allowing them to provide support that is outside the scope of traditional resuscitation algorithms, such as advanced cardiac life support (ACLS).[3,4]

The anesthesiologist plays a critical role in managing both intraoperative and immediate postoperative cardiac arrests. Formulation of a differential diagnosis and rapid application of interventions aimed at the underlying cause of the arrest are essential

[a] Memorial Healthcare System Anesthesiology Residency Program, Envision Physician Services, 703 North Flamingo Road, Pembroke Pines, FL 33028, USA; [b] Envision Physician Services, 7700 W Sunrise Boulevard, Plantation, FL 33322, USA; [c] University of Arizona College of Medicine-Phoenix, 475 N 5th Street, Phoenix, AZ 85004, USA; [d] Division of Surgery and Interventional Sciences, University of College London, Centre for Perioperative Medicine, Charles Bell House, 43-45 Foley Street, London, WIW 7TS, England; [e] Quick'r Care, 990 Biscayne Boulevard #501, Miami, FL 33132, USA
* Corresponding author.
E-mail address: gmaccioli@mac.com

Anesthesiology Clin 38 (2020) 859–873
https://doi.org/10.1016/j.anclin.2020.08.011
1932-2275/20/© 2020 Elsevier Inc. All rights reserved.
anesthesiology.theclinics.com

to optimizing outcomes. Practicing anesthesiologists should have standard procedures that allow for the immediate assessment and management of cardiac arrest in the perioperative environment. This article discusses precardiac arrest considerations, approaches to perioperative crisis and cardiac arrest management, triggers of high-stakes perioperative cardiac arrest (POCA), and therapeutic approaches to these high-stakes arrest scenarios in adult surgical patients.

INCIDENCE, OUTCOMES, AND RISK FACTORS OF PERIOPERATIVE CARDIAC ARREST

POCA is a complication associated with high morbidity and mortality.[5–10] Optimal outcome depends on knowledge of the patient's comorbidities and underlying pathophysiology, recognition of predisposing factors, early detection, aggressive resuscitation, and intensive postresuscitation care. Data obtained between 2010 and 2013 by the National Anesthesia Clinical Outcomes Registry demonstrate that intraoperative cardiac arrests occur in 5.6 per 10,000 patients, with an associated mortality of 58.4%.[11] A more recent study evaluated ICD-10 codes for OR procedures in 2016.[12] They estimated an incidence of 5.7 per 10,000 cases with an in-hospital mortality of 35.7%. Another study in Chile used hospital registry data to show that POCA occurred in 4.4 per 10,000 patients.[13] Patients who developed POCA had a higher survival rate than other types of cardiac arrest, particularly if anesthesia was a contributing factor.

Patients undergoing emergency surgery, those with high American Society of Anesthesiologists physical status scores, and those at the extremes of age have the highest incidence of POCA.[5–10] Additional risk factors include cardiac, vascular or thoracic surgery; congestive heart failure, peripheral vascular disease, end-stage renal disease, pulmonary circulation disorders, and fluid and electrolyte disorders.[13]

UNIQUE CONTRIBUTORS TO PERIOPERATIVE CARDIAC ARREST

POCA frequently involves factors that are not explicitly discussed in conventional ACLS algorithms.[1–4] These include hypoxia associated with difficult airway management; perioperative hemorrhage or hypovolemia; hemodynamic instability due to iatrogenic pneumothorax, pericardial, or abdominal tamponade; circulatory collapse due to auto-positive end-expiratory pressure (auto-PEEP) or inhalational anesthetic overdose; vagal responses to surgical manipulation; and sympatholysis from anesthetic agents, beta-blockers, or neuraxial anesthesia.[14–17] Several high-stakes clinical scenarios can also lead to POCA. These include severe anaphylaxis, systemic local anesthetic toxicity, malignant hyperthermia, severe hyperkalemia, hypertensive crisis, pulmonary embolism, and trauma.[2]

RECOGNITION OF PERIOPERATIVE CRISIS

Anesthesia providers must maintain a high index of suspicion that a crisis is either about to occur or is already occurring. However, many pitfalls impede the recognition of crisis within the perioperative environment.[14,15,18] These include the inability to identify mental status changes due to sedation or general anesthesia; inability to detect tachypnea, hypopnea, or apnea during mechanical ventilation; lack of urine production due to surgically elevated antidiuretic hormone; lack of patient access due to surgical draping and positioning; and environmental factors such as dimly lit ORs and ambient noise. Noise pollution is of particular concern because it may reduce the ability of the anesthesiologist to hear alarms, detect arrhythmias, or recognize deterioration in vital signs.[19]

STEPWISE APPROACH TO THE PERIOPERATIVE PATIENT IN CRISIS
General Considerations

A general approach to the perioperative patient in crisis is outlined in **Fig. 1**. In addition to calling for additional help and equipment, such as a cognitive aid, defibrillator, and ultrasound machine, the anesthesia provider should initiate cardiopulmonary support, communicate with the OR team, and assess whether it is appropriate to stop the procedure. At this time, it is also important to assess monitors, confirm airway integrity/patency, and review recently administered medications and end-tidal carbon dioxide (E_TCO_2) trends. The following sections outline important steps in the management of perioperative prearrest crisis.

Escalation of Monitoring

During crisis, escalation of patient monitoring is nearly always required to guide management. The decision to place additional monitors depends on patient history, underlying pathology and pathophysiology, current clinical status, anesthetic technique, and the surgical procedure being performed.[1–4] Unstable patients should be monitored with an arterial line and care determined by serial arterial blood gas evaluations, including assessments of oxygenation, ventilation, base deficit, and lactate levels. Monitoring via central venous access is reasonable and appropriate when knowledge of central pressures and central venous oxygen saturations might help guide

Communicate Crisis **Initiate cardiopulmonary support** **Obtain equipment**	• Inform team in room of crisis and consider stopping procedure • Call for help, code cart, ultrasound, cognitive aids, other equipment • Check monitors and circuit • Evaluate for cardiac arrest (EKG, pulse, capnography, a-line, oximetry, etc); if appropriate, begin CPR (rate 100–120/min and EtCO2 >20 mm Hg, diastolic BP >40 mm Hg) • Administer empiric vasopressor therapy • Confirm patent airway or consider intubation; increase FiO2
Review data **Obtain testing/imaging** **Generate Differential Diagnosis**	• Follow ACLS algorithms while generating differential diagnosis • Place invasive monitors as indicated; consider non-invasive monitoring • Review end tidal CO2 data before and during event • Review medications and details of procedure / event with team • Obtain testing and imaging (CXR, TEE, POCUS, EKG, etc.) to rule in or out causes
Initiate Targeted Therapy	• Resuscitate based on invasive or non-invasive monitoring • Optimize oxygenation and ventilation settings; minimize auto-PEEP • Implement therapy based on underlying cause of crisis; note that some causes may require specific therapies outside of ACLS algorithms • For LV shock, begin inotropic support (systolic dysfunction) or lusitropic support (diastolic dysfunction); consider IABP, LVAD or ECMO • For RV shock, consider inotropic support, systemic arterial vasoconstrictors, and pulmonary arterial vasodilators; consider RVAD, ECMO

Fig. 1. Approach to the perioperative patient in crisis. After informing the team of the change in clinical condition, it is important to begin cardiopulmonary support (including ACLS) and obtain necessary materials and equipment. Subsequent efforts should be focused on obtaining information to generate a differential diagnosis and begin goal-directed therapy based on available data. The order of actions within each section may vary depending on the clinical scenario.

resuscitation or when providers anticipate the need for catecholamine or inotropic therapies. Transesophageal echocardiography is particularly useful for real-time assessment of cardiac function and volume status.[20,21] If available, the application of continuous noninvasive measures of arterial blood pressure and/or cardiac perfor-mance may be considered as a bridge while placing invasive monitors. Recently, cli-nicians have also increasingly used point of care ultrasound for quick diagnoses and crisis management decisions.[22,23]

Circulatory Support

As indicated earlier, sudden severe perioperative hypotension and/or cardiac arrest may occur for several reasons. Volume status, cardiac function (rate, rhythm, contrac-tility), and systemic tone must be evaluated. Hypovolemia is the most common cause of perioperative hypotension, circulatory crisis, and shock. Under the correct condi-tions, dynamic indices including pulse pressure variation, systolic pressure variation, stroke volume variation, and plethysmographic variability index are strong indicators of volume responsiveness in hypotensive patients.[24-26] These indices are most reli-able in intubated, mechanically ventilated patients who are synchronous with the ventilator (tidal volume ≥ 8 cc/kg) and who have a regular r-r interval. Although contro-versial, dynamic indices may be used to assess volume responsiveness in coopera-tive, spontaneously breathing patients.[27-29] Hypotension in association with a dynamic indices of less than 10%, all conditions met, suggests that hypotension and shock will not improve with fluid resuscitation. Critically, one cannot rule out hypo-volemic hypotension in the setting of "gray zone" range dynamic indices.[30] In this setting, other methods of assessing volume responsiveness, such as a classic volume challenge, must be considered.[31]

Euvolemic hypotensive patients without cardiac failure will often benefit from titrated boluses of vasoactive drugs (ie, phenylephrine, ephedrine, vasopressin, norepinephrine, and epinephrine). Small boluses of vasopressin (0.5–2 Units intrave-nously [IV]) will frequently improve hemodynamics when escalating bolus doses of cat-echolamines have failed.[32,33] In addition, vasopressin administration should be considered for hypotensive vasoplegia in the setting of angiotensin II receptor blockers and angiotensin-converting enzyme inhibitor exposure.[34] Methylene blue has been used successfully in the management of cardiopulmonary bypass-associated hypotensive vasoplegia.[35] The role that angiotensin II might play in unsta-ble perioperative patients has yet to be defined.

Management of Ventricular Shock

Left ventricular failure is another common cause of circulatory crisis. Echocardiogra-phy and invasive monitors, such as a pulmonary artery catheter, should be used to assess cardiac function and guide management.[36,37] In most cases, hypotensive euvolemic patients with left ventricular shock are managed with inotropic agents. Pa-tients with significant diastolic dysfunction may benefit from lusitropic agents, such as milrinone, that enhance ventricular relaxation and improve cardiac output. Impor-tantly, although milrinone may enhance coronary blood flow, it may also reduce sys-temic tone requiring the addition of a catecholamine, such as norepinephrine. Mechanical support with intraaortic balloon pumps, ventricular assist devices, and extracorporeal membrane oxygenation (ECMO) are being increasingly used in hospi-talized patients with severe left ventricular shock.[38-40]

The evaluation and management of right ventricular (RV) shock is best guided using a combination of invasive monitors, such as a pulmonary artery catheter and/or echo-cardiography.[36,37] In most instances, an acute increase in pulmonary vascular resistance (often in the setting of a chronic cause of pulmonary hypertension) causes and sustains RV shock. A combination of inotropes, systemic arterial vasoconstrictors, and pulmonary artery vasodilators such as nitric oxide are used to manage these patients.[41,42] Salvageable patients with RV shock refractory to medical management are increasingly being rescued with mechanical support including ECMO and ventricular assist devices.

Optimization of Oxygenation and Ventilation

Current guidelines recommend avoiding hyperventilation during resuscitation.[43,44] Studies of ventilation during shock repeatedly demonstrate that the duration of increased intrathoracic pressure is proportional to the ventilatory rate, tidal volume, and inspiratory time. Because positive pressure ventilation decreases venous return, and hypoventilation seems to cause no harm, patients in shock should be ventilated with the lowest settings compatible with an oxygen saturation of 90%.[1–4,43,44]

Mechanical ventilation settings must be adjusted to mitigate auto-PEEP. This phenomenon, which is also known as gas trapping or intrinsic PEEP, occurs most commonly in patients with obstructive lung disease.[45] In these patients, mechanical ventilation that does not allow sufficient time for complete exhalation produces a gradual accumulation of air (volume) and an associated increase in pressure (end-expiratory pressure) within the alveoli. This pressure is transmitted to the pulmonary capillaries and decreases both venous return and cardiac output. The presence of auto-PEEP can be inferred whenever the expiratory flow waveform does not return to the zero baseline between breaths.[46,47] Patients at risk for auto-PEEP are best ventilated with the least tolerable tidal volume and rate. Small tidal volumes (<6 mL/kg), a low respiratory rate (<10/min), and a short inspiratory time (1.2–2 seconds) will produce the lowest risk of auto-PEEP–associated circulatory depression, albeit with an increase in peak inspiratory pressure.[48]

UNIQUE FEATURES OF PERIOPERATIVE CARDIAC ARREST

Recognition of cardiac arrest in the OR is not always straightforward.[1–4,18,19] Hemodynamic perturbations deemed abnormal in traditional resuscitation algorithms are frequently encountered during anesthesia. Inconsistent or unreliable monitoring as well as false alarms from electrocardiogram or oximetry may further delay recognition of cardiac arrest.[49] Examples of monitoring difficulties include an improperly damped waveform or wrongly leveled transducer; electrical interference; limitations due to surgical field, body habitus, or positioning; hypothermia; hypovolemia; burn injury; or vasculopathy.

Loss of E_TCO_2 with loss of plethysmograph or arterial line tracing is common in POCA, and evaluation of E_TCO_2 trends should guide both differential diagnosis and interventions.[1–4] Once POCA is confirmed, cardiopulmonary resuscitation (CPR) should be initiated immediately with monitoring of E_TCO_2 to evaluate CPR quality (goal E_TCO_2 >20 mm Hg).[1–4,43,44] Several scenarios that can lead to POCA, along with cause-specific approaches to treatment, are described in the following section (**Fig. 2**).

Severe Anaphylaxis

Anaphylaxis is an immune-mediated hypersensitivity reaction whose severity ranges from minor to life-threatening.[50] The overall incidence seems to be around 15 in 10,000 operations, with severe cases occurring in approximately 2 per 10,000 operations. Initial symptoms are frequently nonspecific, and bronchospasm is not always

	Pneumo-thorax	Pulmonary Embolism	Hypertensive Crisis	Severe Hyperkalemia	Malignant Hyperthermia	LAST	Severe Anaphylaxis
Initial Management (Note that medication doses are guidelines and must be based on patient physiology)	If unstable, perform needle thoracostomy If stable, perform tube thoracostomy	Stop infusion of gas or ask surgeon to flood surgical field FiO2 1.0 Intubate for respiratory distress or refractory hypoxemia Consider Trendelenberg and left lateral decubitus position Consider CPB and emergent thrombectomy	Deepen anesthetic and administer anti-hypertensive medications Place patient in reverse trendelenberg position If appropriate, stop surgery	Administer calcium chloride 1g IV or gluconate Administer 1 ampule D50 and Insulin 10 Units IV Consider 50 mEq NaHCO3 IV and albuterol via ETT Administer furosemide 20–40 mg IV; increase to 1–1.5 mg/kg if no response Consider 30–60 g kayexelate OG/NG/PR Consider washed pRBC Consider ECMO	Discontinue volatile anesthetic Switch from anesthesia ventilator to manual ventilation with separate oxygen source Stop procedure if possible Administer dantrolene 2.5 mg/kg, followed by infusion Start active cooling to 38C with ice packs	Cease administration of local anesthetic Intubate and provide FiO2 1.0 20% lipid emulsion 1.5 mL/kg load then 0.25 mL/kg/min Treat seizures with benzodiazepine Treat symptomatic bradycardia with transcutaneous or intravenous pacemaker If ACLS initiated, consider low dose epinephrine (10–100 mcg IV) and NaHCO3 prn to maintain pH > 7.25; Consider amiodarone, H1 / H2 blocker and ECMO	Stop or remove inciting agent or drug Stop procedure Monitor arterial BP Intubate and administer FiO2 1.0 Administer epinephrine 100–300 mcg IV in escalating doses Consider 2U vasopression, H1 blocker, H2 blocker, corticosteroid, epinephrine infusion If auto-PEEP suspected, adjust ventilator settings Consider ECMO
Subsequent Management	If pneumothorax due to lung injury, consider thoracic surgery	Consider Right ventricular shock algorithm	Monitor for recurrence; address circulatory collapse with CPR	Monitor and treat serum potassium	Monitor for 72 h and treat as necessary; consider muscle biopsy post-crisis	Monitor for recurrence or delayed progression	Determine blood trypase levels within hours; monitor for at least 24 h

Fig. 2. Management of high-stakes perioperative scenarios. The upper row describes initial management steps of each high-stakes scenario. The lower row describes additional management considerations important for optimal patient outcome. (*Adapted from* Maccioli, G. ASA Refresher Course Lecture 2019. With permission.)

present.[51,52] When symptoms of distributive shock develop, moderate doses of epinephrine (100–300 mcg IV) should be administered to halt mast cell degranulation and maintain systolic blood pressure greater than 90 mm Hg. Repeated treatment with escalating doses of epinephrine and initiation of an infusion (0.05–0.3 mcg/kg/min) are frequently required.[53–56] Because laryngeal edema can develop quickly, these patients should be intubated and monitored carefully for auto-PEEP.[52] After stabilization, the patient should be monitored in an intensive care unit (ICU) for at least 24 hours due to a high incidence of recrudescence. Tryptase testing is indicated for diagnostic purposes.

Tension Pneumothorax

Pathologic increases in intrapleural and intrathoracic pressure, as a consequence of air that leaks in via a "one-way" valve can be deadly.[57] This complication is especially concerning in patients receiving positive pressure ventilation because increased intrapleural pressure throughout the respiratory cycle produces a marked decrease in venous return, reduced cardiac output, hypotension, tachycardia, hypoxemia, and if uncorrected, cardiac arrest (pulseless electrical activity [PEA]).[58,59] Immediate management includes treatment with 100% oxygen and the insertion of a thoracostomy tube or large bore peripheral IV catheter in the midclavicular line at the second intercostal space.[60,61]

Local Anesthetic Systemic Toxicity

This life-threatening reaction results when local anesthetic reaches toxic systemic circulating levels. Patients with local anesthetic systemic toxicity (LAST) may demonstrate a range of neurologic and/or cardiovascular symptoms that can be delayed more than 5 minutes from injection of local anesthetic.[62–64] Neurologic symptoms include a metallic taste and/or tinnitus at low levels of toxicity; agitation, obtundation, and seizures occur at higher plasma levels of local anesthetic. Cardiovascular complications may include hypertension and tachycardia, ventricular arrhythmias, as well as progressive hypotension and bradycardia.

The initial treatment of LAST includes ensuring adequate oxygenation, ventilation, and treatment of seizure with a benzodiazepine. Infusion of a 20% lipid emulsion may reduce the chance of cardiovascular complications by reducing peak plasma levels of local anesthetic.[65,66] If LAST progresses to cardiovascular collapse, high-quality CPR will distribute the intralipid throughout the body. Prolonged CPR may be necessary. Reduced doses of epinephrine (<1 mcg/kg) and early consideration of ECMO have been shown to improve outcomes.[65,66] Patients should be monitored in ICU for at least 6 hours following ROSC, as recrudescence of cardiovascular instability can occur.[67]

Malignant Hyperthermia

Malignant hyperthermia (MH) is a rare life-threatening condition (incidence 0.2–1.6 in 100,000) triggered by exposure to volatile anesthetics (halothane, enflurane, isoflurane, desflurane, or sevoflurane) or succinylcholine.[68–70] In susceptible patients, these agents induce an uncontrolled hypermetabolic state resulting in a dramatic increase in oxygen consumption, CO_2 production, and hyperthermia. Early signs of MH include hypercapnia and sinus tachycardia; later signs include muscle rigidity, hyperthermia, and tachypnea.[71] Blood gas analyses often reveal both respiratory and metabolic acidosis.

Rapid identification of MH, discontinuation of triggering agents, and prompt administration of dantrolene (2.5 mg/kg IV) reduce MH mortality from 80% to 1.4%. If a procedure cannot be stopped safely, a nontriggering anesthetic should be instituted, along with oxygen uncontaminated with volatile anesthetics from a separate source. In addition, the team should consult with MH resources (www.mhaus.org or www.emhg.org), and efforts should be made to keep patient temperature at or less than 38°C.[68] Rhabdomyolysis following MH frequently causes renal failure and hyperkalemia. Cooling and monitoring in the ICU should be continued postoperatively for at least 72 hours due to risk of recrudescence.

Severe Hyperkalemia

Hyperkalemia is a potentially lethal electrolyte disturbance.[72,73] Common causes include acidosis, renal pathology, and drug therapy, including the administration of large volumes of packed red blood cells.[73] Patients with severe hyperkalemia may experience bradycardia, hypotension, electrocardiographic changes with peaked T-waves, QRS widening, diminished P waves, and a range of arrhythmias, including atrioventricular blocks, ventricular tachycardia, and ventricular fibrillation.[74–78] Neurologic manifestations of hyperkalemia include muscular weakness and respiratory failure due to flaccid muscle paralysis.[79]

Treatment with beta-2 agonists, such as albuterol, as well as glucose with insulin can be initiated to promote intracellular potassium shift.[80–82] If electrocardiographic changes are present, administration of calcium as a membrane stabilizer is recommended. Treatment with loop diuretics is appropriate in patients with kidney function, whereas renal replacement therapy may be required for those without. If medication-resistant hyperkalemia is considered reversible, therapy with extracorporeal life support is appropriate.

Hypertensive Crisis

Severe increases in arterial blood pressure may lead to cardiovascular and neurologic complications. Intraoperative hypertension is common and easily treated; however, prolonged hypertension may lead to organ dysfunction and poor outcomes.[83,84] Causes of hypertensive crisis include excessive surgical stimulation, aortic cross-clamping, light anesthesia, airway compromise, hypertension due to withdrawal of antihypertensive medications, endobronchial intubation, and hypercarbia. If hypertension proves difficult to manage, the differential diagnosis should be expanded to include less common triggers, such as pheochromocytoma, hyperthyroidism, malignant hyperthermia, elevated intracranial pressure, carcinoid syndrome, autonomic dysreflexia from spinal cord injury, and increased circulatory volume.[83,84]

Pulmonary Embolism

Thromboembolism, venous gas embolism, and fat embolism are the most common causes of perioperative pulmonary embolism.[85,86] In the obstetric population, amniotic fluid embolism is a rare but catastrophic cause of pulmonary embolism.[87] Signs of pulmonary embolism include unexplained hypotension with concurrent decrease in E_tCO_2; desaturation that is only moderately responsive to increased F_iO_2; transitory bronchospasm with increased airway resistance; rapid changes of heart rhythm (often dysrhythmias or bradycardia after a transitory tachycardia); unexplained increase of central venous pressure or all pulmonary pressures; and rapid progression to cardiac arrest (usually PEA).[1-4,88]

Thromboembolism causes circulatory crisis via a combination of mechanical obstruction and the release of inflammatory mediators, which increase RV afterload.[41,42] In severe cases, pulmonary vascular resistance is so great that the right ventricle is unable to maintain output. As the RV fails, it typically dilates, and the interventricular septum flattens and shifts toward the left ventricle further impeding left filling, thus decreasing left ventricular output.

Acute thromboembolism causes cardiac arrest in approximately 5% of cases.[84,85] Echocardiography will typically reveal RV dilatation, dysfunction, and an underfilled left ventricle.[89] The management of thromboembolism depends on the procedure and patient. Therapeutic options range from supportive measures to anticoagulation, thrombolysis, operative thrombectomy, and ECMO.[40,90,91]

As thromboembolism, gas embolism may lead to POCA. Conscious patients who suffer gas embolism can have breathlessness and can develop continuous cough. Other features include arrhythmias, myocardial ischemia, acute hypotension with loss of E_TCO_2, and PEA.[92] Management includes inhibition of further gas entrainment, removal of RV "air-lock" if present, and hemodynamic support focused on improving RV function. Patients undergoing procedures with high risk for gas embolism, such as posterior fossa craniotomy in the sitting position, should be monitored using right parasternal precordial Doppler[93] or transesophageal echocardiography.[20,21,89]

Traumatic Cardiac Arrest

POCA in the setting of trauma is associated with high mortality.[94] Traumatic cardiac arrest (TCA) may occur due to hemorrhage, vasodilatory hypotension, cardiac trauma (acute pericardial tamponade, ischemia, penetrating trauma), hypoxia, acidosis, electrolyte disturbance, nerve reflex, drug usage, anesthetic technique, and/or the procedure being performed.[95-97] Treatment of TCA is a team sport, with all measures carried out concurrently rather than sequentially. Success comes from rapid diagnosis and targeted treatment.

If TCA is caused by hypovolemia, the treatment objective is to achieve immediate hemostasis and reestablish euvolemia.[98–100] It is significantly easier to stop bleeding than it is to replace active blood loss. Compressible external hemorrhage should be managed with direct or indirect pressure, tourniquets, and topical hemostatic agents.[98,101] Noncompressible hemorrhage is more difficult; external splints/pressure, blood products, intravenous fluids, and tranexamic acid maybe necessary until surgical control is achieved. A more detailed discussion of the management of traumatic cardiac arrest is beyond the scope of this article.

Subsequent management of TCA will include damage control resuscitation, which combines permissive hypotension and hemostatic resuscitation with damage control surgery.[102–106] Permissive hypotension allows IV fluid administration to a volume sufficient to maintain a radial pulse and aiming for a systolic blood pressure of 80 to 90 mm Hg. Hemostatic resuscitation is an early use of blood products to prevent exsanguination, dilution of hemostatic blood components, and trauma-induced coagulopathy. Tranexamic acid increases survival from traumatic hemorrhage and is incorporated into many TCA protocols.[105]

SUMMARY AND FUTURE DIRECTIONS

Perioperative crises and POCA, although often catastrophic, are frequently managed in a timely and directed manner because practitioners have a deep knowledge of the patient's medical condition and details of recent procedures. These factors, combined with access to critical monitoring and pharmacologic tools, give the anesthesiologist the ability to prevent progression from crisis to arrest and rescue patients who do arrest. It is hoped that the approaches described here, along with approaches for the rapid identification and management of specific high-stakes clinical scenarios, will help anesthesiologists continue to improve patient outcomes.

CLINICS CARE POINTS

- Intraoperative cardiac arrest is associated with high morbidity and mortality, but has a higher survival rate than other types of arrest, particularly in patients receiving anesthesia.
- Early recognition of intraoperative cardiac arrest may be challenging due to both environmental factors in the procedure suite and physiologic perturbations induced by anesthesia and surgery.
- Once intraoperative cardiac arrest is recognized, rapid evaluation and targeted intervention should be initiated based on the underlying clinical situation as well as knowledge of patient's physiology.
- Anesthesiologists should be familiar with specific perioperative causes of arrest, including hemorrhage/trauma, anaphylaxis, embolism, malignant hyperthermia, hyperkalemia, severe hypertension, pneumothorax, and local anesthetic toxicity.

REFERENCES

1. Moitra VK, Einav S, Thies K-C, et al. Cardiac arrest in the operating room: resuscitation and management for the anesthesiologist: Part 1. Anesth Analg 2018; 126:876–88.

2. McEvoy MD, Thies K-C, Einav S, et al. Cardiac arrest in the operating room : Part 2—special situations in the perioperative period. Anesth Analg 2018;126: 889–903.

3. Truhlár A, Deakin CD, Soar J, et al. Cardiac arrest in special circumstances section collaborators. European resuscitation council guidelines for resuscitation 2015: section 4. Cardiac arrest in special circumstances. Resuscitation 2015; 95:148–201.
4. Moitra VK, Gabrielli A, Maccioli GA, et al. Anesthesia advanced circulatory life support. Can J Anaesth 2012;59:586–603.
5. Sprung J, Warner ME, Contreras MG, et al. Predictors of survival following cardiac arrest in patients undergoing noncardiac surgery: a study of 518,294 patients at a tertiary referral center. Anesthesiology 2003;99:259–69.
6. Li G, Warner M, Lang BH, et al. Epidemiology of anesthesia-related mortality in the United States, 1999-2005. Anesthesiology 2009;110:759–65.
7. Mercedes Aguirre CM, Mayanz SM, Blanch AZ, et al. Registry of perioperative cardiac arrests in a clinical hospital in the period 2006-2017. Rev Med Chil 2019; 147:34–40.
8. Kazaure HS, Roman SA, Rosenthal RA, et al. Cardiac arrest among surgical patients: an analysis of incidence, patient characteristics, and outcomes in ACS-NSQIP. JAMA Surg 2013;148:14–21.
9. Ramachandran SK, Mhyre J, Kheterpal S, et al. American heart association's get with the guidelines-resuscitation investigators. Predictors of survival from perioperative cardiopulmonary arrests: a retrospective analysis of 2,524 events from the get with the guidelines-resuscitation registry. Anesthesiology 2013; 119:1322–39.
10. Fielding-Singh V, Willingham MD, Fischer MA, et al. A population-based analysis of intraoperative cardiac arrest in the United States. Anesth Analg 2020;130: 627–34.
11. Nunnally ME, O'Connor MF, Kordylewski H, et al. The incidence and risk factors for perioperative cardiac arrest observed in the national anesthesia clinical outcomes registry. Anesth Analg 2015;120:364–70.
12. Newland MC, Ellis SJ, Lydiatt CA, et al. Anesthetic-related cardiac arrest and its mortality: a report covering 72,959 anesthetics over 10 years from a US teaching hospital. Anesthesiology 2002;97:108–15.
13. Braz LG, Módolo NS, do Nascimento P Jr, et al. Perioperative cardiac arrest: a study of 53,718 anaesthetics over 9 yr from a Brazilian teaching hospital. Br J Anaesth 2006;96:569–75.
14. Taenzer AH, Pyke JB, McGrath SP. A review of current and emerging approaches to address failure-to-rescue. Anesthesiology 2011;115:421–31.
15. Silber JH, Williams SV, Krakauer H, et al. Hospital and patient characteristics associated with death after surgery. A study of adverse occurrence and failure to rescue. Med Care 1992;30:615–29.
16. Pollard JB. Cardiac arrest during spinal anesthesia: common mechanisms and strategies for prevention. Anesth Analg 2001;92:252–6.
17. Kopp SL, Horlocker TT, Warner ME, et al. Cardiac arrest during neuraxial anesthesia: frequency and predisposing factors associated with survival. Anesth Analg 2005;100:855–65.
18. Wen LY, Howard SK. Perioperative ACLS/Cognitive aids in resuscitation. Int Anesthesiol Clin 2017;55:4–18.
19. Bretonnier M, Michinov E, Morandi X, et al. Interruptions in Surgery: a comprehensive review. J Surg Res 2020;247:190–6.
20. Memtsoudis SG, Rosenberger P, Loffler M, et al. The usefulness of transesophageal echocardiography during intraoperative cardiac arrest in noncardiac surgery. Anesth Analg 2006;102:1653–7.

21. Parker BK, Salerno A, Eurele BD. The use of transesophageal echocardiography during cardiac arrest resuscitation: a literature review. J Ultrasound Med 2019;38:1141–51.

22. Feissel M, Michard F, Faller P, et al. The respiratory variation in inferior vena cava diameter as a guide to fluid therapy. Intensive Care Med 2004;30:1834–7.

23. Breitkreutz R, Walcher F, Seeger FH. Focused echocardiographic evaluation in resuscitation management: concept of an advanced life support-conformed algorithm. Crit Care Med 2007;35(5 suppl):S150–61.

24. Hong DM, Lee JM, Seo JH, et al. Pulse pressure variation to predict fluid responsiveness in spontaneously breathing patients: tidal vs. forced inspiratory breathing. Anaesthesia 2014;69:717–22.

25. Michard F, Teboul JL. Using heart-lung interactions to assess fluid responsiveness during mechanical ventilation. Crit Care 2000;4:282–9.

26. Pizov R, Eden A, Bystritski D, et al. Arterial and plethysmographic waveform analysis in anesthe- tized patients with hypovolemia. Anesthesiology 2010; 113:83–91.

27. Zöllei E, Bertalan V, Németh A, et al. Non-invasive detection of hypovolemia or fluid responsiveness in spontaneously breathing subjects. BMC Anesthesiol 2013;13:40.

28. Bloomstone JA, Nathanson MH, McGee WT. Dynamic indices: use with caution in spontaneously breathing patients. Anesth Analg 2018;127:e47–8.

29. Wyler von Ballmoos M, Takala J, Roeck M, et al. Pulse-pressure variation and hemodynamic response in patients with elevated pulmonary artery pressure: a clinical study. Crit Care 2010;14:R111.

30. Magder S. Clinical usefulness of respiratory variations in arterial pressure. Am J Respir Crit Care Med 2004;169:151–5.

31. Boulain T, Achard JM, Teboul JL, et al. Changes in BP induced by passive leg raising predict response to fluid loading in critically ill patients. Chest 2002;121:1245–52.

32. Müllner M, Urbanek B, Havel C, et al. Vasopressors for shock. Cochrane Database Syst Rev 2004;3:CD003709.

33. Robin JK, Oliver JA, Landry DW. Vasopressin deficiency in the syndrome of irreversible shock. J Trauma 2003;54:S149–54.

34. Bradic N, Povsic-Cevra Z. Surgery and discontinuation of angiotensin converting enzyme inhibitors: current perspectives. Curr Opin Anaesthesiol 2018;31(1):50–4. Available at: https://www.ncbi.nlm.nih.gov/pubmed/29206698.

35. Shah R, Wenger RK, Patel PA, et al. Severe vasoplegic shock during coronary artery bypass surgery: therapeutic challenges and dilemmas in hemodynamic rescue. J Cardiothorac Vasc Anesth 2020;34(5):1341–7. Available at:https://www.ncbi.nlm.nih.gov/pubmed/32146101.

36. Reynolds HR, Hochman JS. Cardiogenic shock: current concepts and improving outcomes. Circulation 2008;117:686–97.

37. Topalian S, Ginsberg F, Parrillo JE. Cardiogenic shock. Crit Care Med 2008;36(1 suppl):S66–74.

38. Shekar K, Mullany DV, Thomson B, et al. Extracorporeal life support devices and strategies for management of acute cardiorespiratory failure in adult patients: a comprehensive review. Crit Care 2014;18:219.

39. Ventetuolo CE, Muratore CS. Extracorporeal life support in critically ill adults. Am J Respir Crit Care Med 2014;190:497–508.

40. Tickoo M, Bardia A. Anesthesia at the edge of life: mechanical circulatory support. Anesthesiol Clin 2020;38:19–33.

41. Haddad F, Doyle R, Murphy DJ, et al. Right ventricular function in cardiovascular disease, part II: pathophysiology, clinical importance, and management of right ventricular failure. Circulation 2008;117:1717–31.

42. Strumpher J, Jacobsohn E. Pulmonary hypertension and right ventricular dysfunction: physiology and perioperative management. J Cardiothorac Vasc Anesth 2011;25:687–704.

43. Kleinman ME, Brennan EE, Goldberger ZD, et al. Part 5: adult basic life support and cardiopulmonary resuscitation quality: 2015 American heart association guidelines update for cardiopulmonary resuscitation and emergency cardiovascular care. Circulation 2015;132:S414–35.

44. Link MS, Berkow LC, Kudenchuk PJ, et al. Part 7: adult advanced cardiovascular life support: 2015 American heart association guidelines update for cardiopulmonary resuscitation and emergency cardiovascular care. Circulation 2015;132:S444–64.

45. Pepe PE, Marini JJ. Occult positive end-expiratory pressure in mechanically ventilated patients with airflow obstruction: the auto-PEEP effect. Am Rev Respir Dis 1982;126:166–70.

46. Franklin C, Samuel J, Hu TC. Life-threatening hypotension associated with emergency intubation and the initiation of mechanical ventilation. Am J Emerg Med 1994;12:425–8.

47. Rogers PL, Schlichtig R, Miro A, et al. Auto-PEEP during CPR. An "occult" cause of electromechanical dissociation? Chest 1991;99:492–3.

48. Adhiyaman V, Adhiyaman S, Sundaram R. The Lazarus phenomenon. J R Soc Med 2007;100:552–7.

49. Tscholl DW, Handschin L, Rossler J, et al. It's not you, it's the design – common problems with patient monitoring reported by anesthesiologists: a mixed qualitative and quantitative study. BMC Anesthesiol 2019;19:87.

50. Neugut AI, Ghatak AT, Miller RL. Anaphylaxis in the United States: an investigation into its epidemiology. Arch Intern Med 2001;161:15–21.

51. Mertes PM, Laxenaire MC. Allergy and anaphylaxis in anaesthesia. Minerva Anestesiol 2004;70:285–91.

52. Saager L, Turan A, Egan C, et al. Incidence of intraoperative hypersensitivity reactions: a registry analysis: a registry analysis. Anesthesiology 2015;122:551–9.

53. Simons FE, Sheikh A. Anaphylaxis: the acute episode and beyond. BMJ 2013;346:f602.

54. Pumphrey RS. Lessons for management of anaphylaxis from a study of fatal reactions. Clin Exp Allergy 2000;30:1144–50.

55. Sheikh A, Shehata YA, Brown SG, et al. Adrenaline (epinephrine) for the treatment of anaphylaxis with and without shock. Cochrane Database Syst Rev 2008;2008(4):CD006312.

56. Korenblat P, Lundie MJ, Dankner RE, et al. A retrospective study of epinephrine administration for anaphylaxis: how many doses are needed? Allergy Asthma Proc 1999;20:383–6.

57. Roberts DJ, Leigh-Smith S, Faris PD, et al. Clinical presentation of patients with tension pneumothorax: a systematic review. Ann Surg 2015;261:1068–78.

58. Leigh-Smith S, Harris T. Tension pneumothorax—time for a rethink? Emerg Med J 2005;22:8–16.

59. Phillips S, Falk GL. Surgical tension pneumothorax during laparoscopic repair of massive hiatus hernia: a different situation requiring different management. Anaesth Intensive Care 2011;39:1120–3.

60. Roberts DJ, Niven DJ, James MT, et al. Thoracic ultrasonography versus chest radiography for detection of pneumothoraces: challenges in deriving and interpreting summary diagnostic accuracy estimates. Crit Care 2014;18:416.
61. Kenny L, Teasdale R, Marsh M, et al. Techniques of training in the management of tension pneumothorax: bridging the gap between confidence and competence. Ann Transl Med 2016;4:233.
62. Weinberg G, Barron G. Local anesthetic systemic toxicity (LAST): not gone, hopefully not forgotten. Reg Anesth Pain Med 2016;41:1–2.
63. Di Gregorio G, Neal JM, Rosenquist RW, et al. Clinical presentation of local anesthetic systemic toxicity: a review of published cases, 1979 to 2009. Reg Anesth Pain Med 2010;35:181–7.
64. Vasques F, Behr AU, Weinberg G, et al. A review of local anesthetic systemic toxicity cases since publication of the American society of regional anesthesia recommendations: to whom it may concern. Reg Anesth Pain Med 2015;40: 698–705.
65. McCutchen T, Gerancher JC. Early intralipid therapy may have prevented bupivacaine-associated cardiac arrest. Reg Anesth Pain Med 2008;33:178–80.
66. Dureau P, Charbit B, Nicolas N, et al. Effect of Intralipid® on the dose of ropivacaine or levobupivacaine tolerated by volunteers: a clinical and pharmacokinetic study. Anesthesiology 2016;125:474–83.
67. Marwick PC, Levin AI, Coetzee AR. Recurrence of cardiotoxicity after lipid rescue from bupivacaine-induced cardiac arrest. Anesth Analg 2009;108: 1344–6.
68. Ellinas H, Albrecht MA. Malignant Hyperthermia update. Anesthesiol Clin 2020; 38:165–81.
69. Ording H. Incidence of malignant hyperthermia in Denmark. Anesth Analg 1985; 64:700–4.
70. Lu Z, Rosenberg H, Brady JE, et al. Prevalence of malignant hyperthermia diagnosis in New York state ambulatory surgery center discharge records 2002 to 2011. Anesth Analg 2016;122:449–53.
71. Larach MG, Brandom BW, Allen GC, et al. Cardiac arrests and deaths associated with malignant hyperthermia in North America from 1987 to 2006: a report from the North American malignant hyperthermia registry of the malignant hyperthermia association of the United States. Anesthesiology 2008;108:603–11.
72. Oh PC, Koh KK, Kim JH, et al. Life threatening severe hyperkalemia presenting typical electrocardiographic changes—rapid recovery following medical, temporary pacing, and hemodialysis treatments. Int J Cardiol 2014;177:27–9.
73. An JN, Lee JP, Jeon HJ, et al. Severe hyperkalemia requiring hospitalization: predictors of mortality. Crit Care 2012;16:R225.
74. Slade TJ, Grover J, Benger J. Atropine-resistant bradycardia due to hyperkalaemia. Emerg Med J 2008;25:611–2.
75. Sohoni A, Perez B, Singh A. Wenckebach block due to hyperkalemia: a case report. Emerg Med Int 2010;2010:879751.
76. Kim NH, Oh SK, Jeong JW. Hyperkalaemia induced complete atrioventricular block with a narrow QRS complex. Heart 2005;91:e5.
77. Tiberti G, Bana G, Bossi M. Complete atrioventricular block with unwidened QRS complex during hyperkalemia. Pacing Clin Electrophysiol 1998;21:1480–2.
78. Yin Y, Zhu T. Ventricular fibrillation during anesthesia in a Wenchuan earthquake victim with crush syndrome. Anesth Analg 2010;110:916–7.
79. Freeman SJ, Fale AD. Muscular paralysis and ventilatory failure caused by hyperkalaemia. Br J Anaesth 1993;70:226–7.

80. Woodforth IJ. Resuscitation from transfusion-associated hyperkalaemic ventricular fibrillation. Anaesth Intensive Care 2007;35:110–3.
81. Depret F, Peacock WF, Liu KD, et al. Management of hyperkalemia in the acutely ill patient. Ann Intensive Care 2019;32:1–16.
82. DeFronzo RA, Felig P, Ferrannini E, et al. Effect of graded doses of insulin on splanchnic and peripheral potassium metabolism in man. Am J Phys 1980; 238:E421–7.
83. Aronson S. Perioperative hypertensive emergencies. Curr Hypertens Rep 2014; 16:448.
84. Klimkina O. Anesthesia and hypertensive emergencies. In: Goudra B, et al, editors. Anesthesiology. Cham (Switzerland): Springer; 2018. p. 535–43.
85. Goldhaber SZ, Visani L, De Rosa M. Acute pulmonary embolism: clinical outcomes in the International cooperative pulmonary embolism registry (ICOPER). Lancet 1999;353:1386–9.
86. Tapson VF. Acute pulmonary embolism. N Engl J Med 2008;358:1037–52.
87. Fardelmann KL, Alian AA. Anesthesia for obstetric disasters. Anesthesiol Clin 2020;38:85–105.
88. Lavonas EJ, Drennan IR, Gabrielli A, et al. Part 10: special circumstances of resuscitation: 2015 American heart association guidelines update for cardiopulmonary resuscitation and emergency cardiovascular care. Circulation 2015; 132:S501–18.
89. Price S, Uddin S, Quinn T. Echocardiography in cardiac arrest. Curr Opin Crit Care 2010;16:211–5.
90. Abu-Laban RB, Christenson JM, Innes GD, et al. Tissue plasminogen activator in cardiac arrest with pulseless electrical activity. N Engl J Med 2002;346: 1522–8.
91. Böttiger BW, Arntz HR, Chamberlain DA, et al. TROICA trial investigators; European resuscitation council study group. Thrombolysis during resuscitation for out-of-hospital cardiac arrest. N Engl J Med 2008;359:2651–62.
92. Mirski MA, Lele AV, Fitzsimmons L, et al. Diagnosis and treatment of vascular air embolism. Anesthesiology 2007;106:164–77.
93. Schubert A, Deogaonkar A, Drummond C. Precordial Doppler probe placement for optimal detection of venous air embolism during craniotomy. Anesth Analg 2006;102:1543–7.
94. Zwingmann J, Mehlhorn AT, Hammer T, et al. Survival and neurologic outcome after traumatic out-of-hospital cardiopulmonary arrest in a pediatric and adult population: a systematic review. Crit Care 2012;16:R117.
95. Leis CC, Hernández CC, Blanco MJ, et al. Traumatic cardiac arrest: should advanced life support be initiated? J Trauma Acute Care Surg 2013;74:634–8.
96. Kleber C, Giesecke MT, Lindner T, et al. Requirement for a structured algorithm in cardiac arrest following major trauma: epidemiology, management errors, and preventability of traumatic deaths in Berlin. Resuscitation 2014;85:405–10.
97. Willis CD, Cameron PA, Bernard SA, et al. Cardiopulmonary resuscitation after traumatic cardiac arrest is not always futile. Injury 2006;37:448–54.
98. Spahn DR, Bouillon B, Cerny V, et al. Management of bleeding and coagulopathy following major trauma: an updated European guideline. Crit Care 2013; 17:R76.
99. Bickell WH, Wall MJ Jr, Pepe PE, et al. Immediate versus delayed fluid resuscitation for hypotensive patients with penetrating torso injuries. N Engl J Med 1994;331:1105–9.

100. Harris T, Thomas GO, Brohi K. Early fluid resuscitation in severe trauma. BMJ 2012;345:e5752.
101. Harris T, Davenport R, Hurst T, et al. Improving outcome in severe trauma: trauma systems and initial management: intubation, ventilation and resuscitation. Postgrad Med J 2012;88:588–94.
102. Jansen JO, Thomas R, Loudon MA, et al. Damage control resuscitation for patients with major trauma. BMJ 2009;338:b1778.
103. Holcomb JB, Tilley BC, Baraniuk S, et al, PROPPR Study Group. Transfusion of plasma, platelets, and red blood cells in a 1:1:1 vs a 1:1:2 ratio and mortality in patients with severe trauma: the PROPPR randomized clinical trial. JAMA 2015; 313:471–82.
104. Eastridge BJ, Salinas J, McManus JG, et al. Hypotension begins at 110 mm Hg: redefining "hypotension" with data. J Trauma 2007;63:291–7.
105. Roberts I, Shakur H, Afolabi A, et al. CRASH-2 Collaborators. The importance of early treatment with tranexamic acid in bleeding trauma patients: an exploratory analysis of the CRASH-2 randomised controlled trial. Lancet 2011;377: 1096–101.
106. Sridhar S, Gumbert SD, Stephens C, et al. Resuscitative endovascular balloon occlusion of the aorta: principles, initial clinical experience, and considerations for the anesthesiologist. Anesth Analg 2017;125:884–90.

The Lost Airway

Paul Potnuru, MD[a], Carlos A. Artime, MD[a], Carin A. Hagberg, MD[b],*

KEYWORDS

• Difficult airway • Failed airway • Cricothyrotomy • Human factors

KEY POINTS

• In the most serious cases, the clinician may encounter a failed airway that results from a failure to ventilate an anesthetized patient via facemask or supraglottic airway or intubate the patient with an endotracheal tube.
• This dreaded cannot intubate, cannot oxygenate situation necessitates emergency invasive access, such as surgical cricothyrotomy or needle cricothyrotomy followed by transtracheal jet ventilation.
• The incidence, management, and complications of the failed airway and training issues related to its management are reviewed.

INTRODUCTION

Management of the unanticipated difficult airway is one of the most relevant and challenging crisis management scenarios encountered in clinical anesthesia practice. Several guidelines and approaches have been developed to assist clinicians in navigating this high-acuity scenario.[1–4] In the most serious cases, the clinician may encounter a failed airway that results from a failure to ventilate an anesthetized patient by any means, including facemask, supraglottic airway (SGA) or endotracheal intubation. This dreaded cannot intubate, cannot oxygenate (CICO) situation necessitates emergency invasive access, such as scalpel cricothyrotomy or needle cricothyrotomy followed by transtracheal jet ventilation (TTJV).

This article reviews the incidence, management, and complications of the failed airway and training issues related to its management.

INCIDENCE OF THE FAILED AIRWAY

With careful planning and a structured approach to airway management, the failed airway should be an extremely rare event. A CICO situation requiring an emergency

a Department of Anesthesiology, McGovern Medical School, University of Texas Health Science Center at Houston, 6431 Fannin Street, MSB 5.020, Houston, TX 77030, USA; b Anesthesiology, Critical Care & Pain Medicine, Department of Anesthesiology and Perioperative Medicine, University of Texas MD Anderson Cancer Center, 1400 Holcombe Boulevard, Unit 409, Houston, TX 77030, USA
* Corresponding author.
E-mail address: chagberg@mdanderson.org

Anesthesiology Clin 38 (2020) 875–888
https://doi.org/10.1016/j.anclin.2020.08.012
1932-2275/20/Published by Elsevier Inc.

anesthesiology.theclinics.com

surgical airway occurs in approximately 1 in 50,000 general anesthesia cases.[5] The failed airway, however, can account for up to 1 in 4 anesthesia-related deaths.

The results of the 4th National Audit Project (NAP4), a 1-year audit that aimed at determining the incidence of major complications of airway management in the United Kingdom, were reported in 2011 by the Royal College of Anaesthetists and the Difficult Airway Society.[6] Out of 133 major airway-related events in the perioperative setting, emergency surgical airway was attempted in 58 (43%) cases. Of these 58 cases, 25 attempts were performed by an anesthesiologist. Among the 58 invasive airway attempts, scalpel cricothyrotomy was used successfully as the initial approach in 3 cases and surgical tracheostomy was the successful initial approach in 29 cases. Needle cricothyrotomy failed in 15 out of 19 initial attempts, which were successfully rescued by scalpel-based techniques in 9 cases. Similarly, scalpel-based techniques were used to rescue 2 out of 3 failed attempts at percutaneous dilational cricothyrotomy.

In a review of 102 malpractice claims of difficult tracheal intubation from the Anesthesia Closed Claims Project (ACCP) database between 2000 and 2012, the investigators found that a CICO situation was encountered in a majority of claims.[7] Furthermore, they identified delays in obtaining a surgical airway in more than one-third of CICO cases, in which care deviated from current guidelines for the management of the failed airway.[1–3]

Results from NAP4 and the ACCP reveal that although the failed airway is a rare event, it can be associated with disastrous consequences, including brain damage, cardiac arrest, and death. The failed airway can account for up to 25% of anesthesia-related mortality.[5] The poor outcomes from a failed airway largely are attributed to failure to perform an emergency surgical airway or a delayed decision to do so.[8] Several factors can contribute to the reluctance to perform an emergency surgical airway, including unfamiliarity with equipment and technique, clinical duress, and complex patients.[9] Rescuing the failed airway with emergency invasive airway access, however, can be performed successfully and safely by anesthesiologists with adequate training.

MANAGEMENT OF THE FAILED AIRWAY

Conceptually, airway access can be divided into noninvasive approaches and invasive infraglottic approaches. Failure of the 3 noninvasive approaches (facemask, supraglottic airway [SGA], and endotracheal intubation) results in a CICO scenario, necessitating invasive infraglottic airway access. Invasive airway management techniques include needle or scalpel cricothyrotomy and surgical tracheostomy. The choice of technique depends on the expertise of the clinician, the availability of equipment and personnel, and technical patient factors.

Prediction and Planning

Anticipation and planning are fundamental principles of crisis management in anesthesiology.[10] The importance of the preoperative airway assessment and careful planning cannot be overemphasized. Results from the ACCP revealed that a majority of patients with claims related to difficult tracheal intubation had predictors of a difficult airway.[7] Furthermore, failure to plan for a difficult airway was a common judgment error identified in the claims analysis. A careful airway history and physical examination to identify potential problems with airway management must be performed when feasible in all patients.[1] Although no single physical examination finding can reliably predict a difficult airway, findings suggestive of a difficult airway can assist with planning of the airway management strategy.[11] Whenever applicable, previous airway management records should be examined, because prior difficult intubation can predict challenging airway management. Any available diagnostic imaging of the airway should be reviewed to assist with planning. Computed tomography and magnetic resonance imaging scans can provide valuable information regarding causes of airway pathology, level and severity of any stenosis or obstruction, or any subglottic extension. A preoperative endoscopic airway examination can be performed by the anesthesiologist at the bedside to examine upper airway anatomy and identify abnormalities that may have an impact on airway management.[12] In patients predicted to have a difficult airway, preemptive identification of the cricothyroid membrane (CTM) by palpation and bedside ultrasonography should be considered.[13] Based on the assessment, the anesthesiologist always should have a carefully planned strategy for airway management prior to the induction of anesthesia. The American Society of Anesthesiologists difficult airway algorithm suggests that the airway practitioner consider the relative merits and feasibility of the following 4 basic airway management strategies[1]:

- Awake intubation versus intubation after induction of general anesthesia
- Preservation versus ablation of spontaneous ventilation
- Video-assisted laryngoscopy as the initial approach to intubation
- Noninvasive techniques versus invasive techniques for the initial approach to airway access

Awakening the Patient

When a failed airway is encountered, rapid recovery of spontaneous ventilation is a desirable goal. There are practical limitations, however, to safely achieving this endpoint in a timely manner after the induction of anesthesia,[14] namely, the reversal of neuromuscular blockade and the reversal of other induction agents that cause respiratory depression. With the introduction of sugammadex into clinical practice, rapid reversal of neuromuscular blockade has been suggested as a potential CICO rescue technique.[15] Sugammadex offers significantly faster recovery from neuromuscular blockade over spontaneous recovery from succinylcholine.[16] In a simulation study, however, the mean time to administration of sugammadex was 6.7 minutes after the identification of a CICO scenario, accounting for the time to obtain the drug and administer it.[17] Even in an ideal-case scenario, in which sugammadex fully reversed the neuromuscular block within 4.5 minutes, if ventilation is inadequate, oxygen desaturation still occurs, especially in obese patients.[14,16] Furthermore, profound reversal with sugammadex has been reported to cause laryngospasm and further impairment of ventilation in CICO scenarios.[18] Finally, despite adequate reversal of neuromuscular blockade, the respiratory depression induced by hypnotics and opioids can delay the return of spontaneous ventilation and patient responsiveness.[14] Therefore, the rescue of a CICO scenario should focus on emergency invasive airway access rather than relying on pharmacologic intervention and awakening of the patient.

INVASIVE AIRWAY ACCESS

Rescuing the airway in a CICO scenario is most likely to be successful if a simple, well-rehearsed technique is performed using standardized equipment. Current evidence indicates that a surgical technique is the best initial approach that meets these criteria.[19–21]

Cricothyrotomy

Cricothyrotomy (also referred to as cricothyroidotomy, cricothyroidostomy, cricothyrostomy, laryngostomy, or laryngotomy) is a procedure that involves placing a tube or catheter through the CTM to establish a patent airway. Cricothyrotomy can be classified into 3 broad techniques: scalpel cricothyrotomy, narrow-bore needle cricothyrotomy, and percutaneous dilational cricothyrotomy.[22] All 3 techniques begin with identification of the CTM.

Anatomy and identification of the cricothyroid membrane

The CTM is a ligament that lies inferior to the thyroid cartilage and superior to the cricoid cartilage. Structures that can overlie the CTM include the cricothyroid artery and vein, the pyramidal lobe of the thyroid gland, and lymph nodes. It is conventionally identified by palpating a notch, slight indentation, or dip in the skin inferior to the laryngeal prominence. The laryngeal handshake technique is recommended over conventional palpation to improve the identification of the midline of the neck and CTM. This technique is performed with the nondominant hand, identifying the hyoid and thyroid laminae with the thumb and middle finger, stabilizing the larynx, and moving down the neck to palpate the CTM with the index finger[23] (**Fig. 1**). Several studies have noted that identification of the CTM is unreliable by physical examination alone and that ultrasonography is superior to palpation.[13,24,25] The utility of ultrasonography, however, to identify the CTM in an emergency situation is limited by the immediate availability of equipment and an operator sufficiently familiar with the ultrasound technique. In patients with a predicted difficult airway or those in whom a physical examination cannot easily identify the CTM, ultrasound identification should be performed during the preinduction assessment, when feasible.[21] You-Ten and colleagues[26] found that practice with ultrasound-guided palpation of neck landmarks improves subsequent identification of the CTM using palpation alone. Once the CTM is successfully identified, it can be accessed either via a scalpel or a needle technique.

Scalpel cricothyrotomy

Although various approaches to scalpel cricothyrotomy exist, none has been shown to be superior to the others.[27] All the approaches have the following steps in common: neck extension, identification of the CTM, incision through the skin and CTM, and

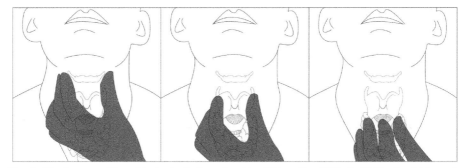

Fig. 1. The laryngeal handshake technique for identifying the CTM. (*left*) The hyoid bone is identified with the thumb and middle finger; (*center*) next, the thyroid cartilage is identified; (*right*) finally, the cricoid cartilage is identified and the index finger is used to identify the cricothyroid membrane. (*From* Oh H, Yoon S, Seo M. Utility of the Laryngeal Handshake Method for Identifying the Cricothyroid Membrane. *Acta Anaesthesiol Scand.* 2018 Oct;62(9):1223-1228; with permission.)

insertion of a cuffed tube. At an institutional level, it is important to have a standardized approach to invasive airway access with readily available equipment, consistent training and skill maintenance programs.[28] This article reviews the scalpel-bougie-tube technique, a simple, fast, and reliable method of providing invasive airway access, which is recommended as the first-line technique by the Difficult Airway Society.[2,29] This technique is performed using minimal equipment that usually is available in a perioperative setting, provides the ability to ventilate using low-pressure ventilation equipment, allows confirmation with capnography, and offers protection from aspiration.

Three pieces of equipment are required for this technique: a number 10 blade scalpel (a broad blade at least as wide as the tracheal tube), a size 6.0-mm cuffed tracheal tube, and a tracheal tube introducer (bougie). In preparation for this technique, operating conditions should be optimized by delivering 100% oxygen to the upper airway, fully extending the neck, and ensuring full neuromuscular blockade. If applicable, manual in-line stabilization should be released to allow full neck extension. Steps to perform the scalpel-bougie-tube technique are outlined in **Box 1** and **Fig. 2**.

If this technique fails due to misidentification of the CTM or the CTM is not easily identified, a more invasive technique to identify the CTM must be employed: make an 8-cm to 10-cm skin vertical incision in the midline of the neck in the caudal to cephalad direction, use blunt dissection with fingers of both hands to separate tissues, identify and stabilize the larynx, identify the CTM, and proceed with the technique, as detailed previously.

This technique is not appropriate as a first-line approach for children younger than 10 years to 12 years of age.[30] They have a small CTM, a narrow airway and a compliant larynx rendering the scalpel technique very challenging. Needle cricothyrotomy should be considered the technique of choice in young infants and children. The presence of an infraglottic obstruction is a relative contraindication because a cricothyrotomy may not bypass the obstruction. Other relative contraindications include laryngeal fracture, laryngotracheal disruption, transection of the trachea, or anatomic distortion of the landmarks.

The complication rate of performing a scalpel cricothyrotomy ranges from 14% to 50% depending on the technique used, the clinical settings, and provider experience.[30,31] The most common complication is venous hemorrhage, which is expected

---

Box 1
Steps to perform a scalpel cricothyrotomy using the scalpel-bougie-tube technique

- Stand on the same side of the patient as the practitioner's dominant hand, which is used to make the incisions.

- If the CTM is easily identifiable, stabilize the larynx with the nondominant hand and use the dominant hand to make a single stab incision horizontally through the CTM with the sharp edge of a number 10 scalpel blade oriented toward the practitioner. Without removing the blade from the incision, turn the scalpel blade 90° so that the sharp edge is oriented caudally.

- Insert a tracheal tube introducer (bougie) into the airway and advance it 10 cm to 15 cm.

- Insert a lubricated 6.0-mm endotracheal tube over the introducer into the airway.

- Inflate the cuff of the endotracheal tube, remove the bougie, and ventilate the patient.

- Confirm the position of the endotracheal tube with capnography, inspection, and auscultation.

- Secure the tracheal tube.

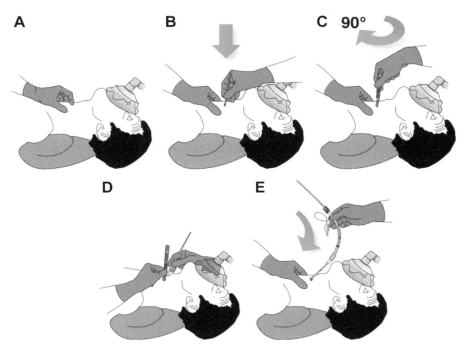

Fig. 2. Scalpel-bougie technique—stab, twist, bougie, and tube. (*A*) The CTM is identified. (*B*) A transverse stab incision is made through the CTM. (*C*) The scalpel is rotated so that the sharp edge points caudally. (*D*) The scalpel is pulled toward the operator to open up the incision, and the coudé tip of the bougie is slid down the scalpel blade into the trachea. (*E*) The endotracheal tube is advanced into the trachea. (*From* Frerk C, Mitchell VS, McNarry AF, et al. Difficult Airway Society 2015 guidelines for management of unanticipated difficult intubation in adults. *Br J Anaesth.* 2015;115(6):827-848; with permission.)

and can be controlled easily with pressure. Major arterial bleeding can occur but usually results from misidentification of the CTM and misplacing the incision. Other early complications include damage to the laryngeal structures, perforation of the trachea, creation of a false tract, and infection.[31] If a patient is ventilated through a misplaced tube (ie, into a false tract), subcutaneous emphysema and distortion of the neck anatomy can occur making subsequent airway management even more challenging. Failure to adequately secure the tube can result in inadvertent extubation.

Needle cricothyrotomy

Needle cricothyrotomy involves percutaneous puncture of the CTM to allow passage of an over-the-needle catheter to facilitate oxygenation. Needle cricothyrotomy can be divided into narrow-bore cricothyrotomy (<4-mm catheter) or percutaneous dilational (>4-mm catheter) cricothyrotomy.

Narrow-bore needle cricothyrotomy Narrow-bore needle cricothyrotomy involves the placement of a narrow-bore catheter (<4 mm) using an over-the-needle technique through the CTM. Once the catheter is in place, this technique requires a specialized high-pressure ventilation source to facilitate low-frequency TTJV.[32]

The equipment required for performing narrow-bore needle cricothyrotomy in adults includes a needle with an overlying catheter (14-gauge) that can be connected to a syringe, a syringe half-filled with saline, oxygen source, high-pressure oxygen tubing, a jet ventilator device, and a 3-way stopcock or Luer lock device. If available, specialized TTJV catheters, which are kink-resistant and curved for easier placement, should be used instead of intravenous catheters. The steps to perform a needle cricothyrotomy and TTJV are outlined in **Box 2**.[29]

Although narrow-bore needle cricothyrotomy is an attractive option for anesthesiologists due to their familiarity with over-the-needle techniques, it is prone to complications that should be considered carefully. Results from NAP4 demonstrated that almost two-thirds of the narrow-bore needle cricothyrotomies performed failed when used as the first attempt at CICO rescue.[6] Common issues included device misplacement, kinking of the catheter, and detachment of the catheter from the ventilation source. A systematic review of narrow-bore needle cricothyrotomy with TTJV in CICO emergencies revealed a high incidence of failure (42%), complications (51%), and barotrauma (32%).[33] Misplacement of the catheter outside the airway and high-pressure ventilation through it can result in rapid development of subcutaneous emphysema. This technique does not provide a tracheal cuff to secure the airway and thus requires conversion to a more definitive airway to protect against aspiration. Familiarity with specialized equipment for TTJV is imperative to the safe execution of this technique.

Percutaneous dilational cricothyrotomy Percutaneous dilation cricothyrotomy uses either a catheter over guidewire (Seldinger technique) or catheter over trocar (without a guide wire) to place a wide-bore catheter (>4 mm) in the airway. The placement of a wide-bore catheter allows for the use of conventional low-pressure ventilation techniques instead of TTJV that is used with narrow-bore needle cricothyrotomy. Additionally, the ability to place a cuffed tube using this technique offers protection from aspiration and allows for positive pressure ventilation.

Commercial cricothyrotomy kits are available that contain all essential equipment to perform percutaneous dilational cricothyrotomy. For example, the Cook Melker kit

---

Box 2
Steps to perform a needle cricothyrotomy and transtracheal jet ventilation

Performing a needle cricothyrotomy
- Identify the CTM and stabilize the larynx with the nondominant hand.
- Hold the syringe attached to the over-the-needle intravenous catheter in the dominant hand.
- Place the catheter in the midline of the neck at the inferior margin of the CTM with the needle oriented caudally at an angle of 30° to 45°.
- Exert downward pressure to puncture through the CTM while applying constant negative pressure to the syringe plunger.
- Stop advancing the needle as soon as entrance into the airway is signaled by bubbles in the saline-containing syringe or air aspiration with minimal effort.
- Hold the needle in place and advance the catheter over the needle and into the airway.
- When the hub of the catheter reaches the skin, remove the needle and use the syringe to aspirate air from the catheter to confirm placement.
- Connect the catheter to an oxygen source.
- Manually hold the catheter in place until a definitive airway is established.

Performing transtracheal jet ventilation
- Connect the catheter to high-pressure tubing.
- Begin regular ventilation using an I:E ratio of 1:4 to 1:5.
- Confirm placement using capnography, chest rise, auscultation, and oxygenation improvement.

includes the following: a scalpel blade, a 6-mL syringe, an 18-gauge needle with an over-the-needle catheter, a guide wire, a dilator, and airway catheters. The insertion procedure for the Cook Melker kit is outlined in **Box 3**.[34]

The use of a wire-guided (Seldinger) technique that is familiar to anesthesiologists presents an attractive option for invasive airway in an emergency CICO situation that is less invasive than a scalpel cricothyrotomy. It also does not require a specialized high-pressure ventilation system unlike the narrow-bore needle cricothyrotomy. Despite the advantages of this technique, results from NAP4 showed a high failure rate (43%) of percutaneous dilational techniques, similar to narrow-bore techniques, that were rescued by scalpel-based techniques.[6] Cadaver studies also have noted longer insertion times in the hands of inexperienced operators.[35] A high incidence of guide wire kinking and device misplacement also has been reported.[36] Some investigators contend, however, that anesthesiologists can safely perform a percutaneous dilational or needle cricothyrotomy as a first-line attempt with adequate training and standardized equipment availability.[28,37]

Surgical Tracheostomy

Tracheostomy is the establishment of a surgical opening in the airway below the cricotracheal membrane (first tracheal ring and below), differing from cricothyrotomy in the anatomic location of airway entry.[38] This technique generally is most familiar to surgeons, in particular trauma surgeons, oral and maxillofacial surgeons, and head and neck surgeons. Head and neck cases account for a large portion of failed

---

Box 3
Steps to perform a percutaneous dilational cricothyrotomy using a Cook Melker kit

- Open the prepackaged cricothyrotomy set and assemble the components. Fill the syringe with 3 mL of saline. Insert the dilator into the airway catheter.

- Position the patient with the neck extended, identify the CTM as above, and stabilize the larynx with the nondominant hand.

- Advance the syringe and the attached 18G introducer needle through the CTM into the airway at a 45° caudad angle while applying constant negative pressure to the syringe plunger.

- Stop advancing the needle as soon as entrance to the airway is signaled by bubbles in the syringe or air aspiration with minimal effort.

- Remove the syringe, leaving the introducer needle in place.

- Advance the soft, flexible end of the guide wire through the needle into the airway.

- Remove the needle, leaving the guide wire in place.

- Make a 1-cm to 2-cm incision through the skin and CTM with the scalpel blade at the entry point of the guide wire.

- Thread the airway catheter and dilator assembly over the guide wire and advance it through the skin incision into the airway following the curve of the dilator.

- Once the airway catheter is flush with the skin, remove the dilator while holding the airway catheter in place.

- Inflate the cuff, if present, and connect the airway catheter to a ventilatory device.

- Confirm placement with capnography, auscultation and chest rise.

- Secure the airway catheter to the neck.

airways.[12] When a surgeon who can perform a surgical tracheostomy is readily available in a CICO emergency, this technique can be performed as effectively and safely as a scalpel cricothyrotomy.[31] Given the need for specialized surgical training and equipment, however, and anatomic challenges associated with emergently accessing the tracheal interspaces, a surgical tracheostomy is not recommended as a first-line attempt at an invasive surgical airway by anesthesiologists.[2,3,29]

Management After Invasive Airway Access

After securing invasive airway access, the ability to successfully oxygenate and ventilate the patient should be verified by clinical exam, capnography, pulse oximetry, and arterial blood gas analysis (when indicated).[39] Inadequate oxygenation or ventilation may require prompt conversion to a more definitive airway. A chest radiograph should be obtained to check for pneumothorax or pneumomediastinum. The patient should be monitored for mediastinal infection given the risk of pharyngeal or esophageal injury from invasive airway access procedures. Surgical consultation to assess and plan for a definitive airway should be made early. Traditional surgical teaching recommends converting a cricothyrotomy to a tracheostomy within 72 hours to prevent subglottic stenosis.[40] The rate of subglottic stenosis, however, with emergency cricothyrotomy may not be significantly higher than with tracheostomy, and existing evidence does not support routine conversion to tracheostomy.[31] When deciding whether to convert the airway, factors to consider include adequacy of gas exchange, the need for prolonged mechanical ventilation, and technical feasibility of conversion to a different airway device.[41] Conversion to a tracheostomy may be better suited to prolonged mechanical ventilation for longer than a week due to a lower risk of clinically significant long-term complications compared with cricothyrotomy.[42]

Management of a failed airway should be thoroughly documented with the intent of informing future care of the patient.[1] Documentation should include detailed descriptions of the specific difficulties encountered and the airway management techniques employed. The patient should be informed of the airway difficulty that was encountered and a written letter or report should be provided for patient and future health care provider reference. The anesthesiologist should report the management of the failed airway to relevant airway databases and registries, which can improve individual patient care and provide research data to advance clinical practice.[43]

Perioperative crises can have profound and long-lasting effects on anesthesiologists and other health care staff involved.[44] Team debriefing should occur after an airway crisis to help mitigate the negative impact of such events, promote learning, and improve patient safety.[45]

HUMAN FACTORS AND TRAINING ISSUES

Much of the literature on airway management since the results of NAP4 were published has focused on the role of human factors in the successful management of CICO emergencies[8,46,47] (see Barbara K. Burian and R. Key Dismukes' article, "Why We Fail to Rescue During Critical Events," in this issue) Analyses of failed attempts at CICO rescue have revealed deficiencies on the individual, team, and organization levels that must be addressed in the implementation of and training for an effective airway management strategy.[6,7]

On an individual level, clinicians involved in an airway emergency are vulnerable to errors from the unproductive cognitive effects of acute stress on attention, memory, and decision making.[48] Although stress can improve selective attention on a given task, it also can diminish situational awareness, leading to errors, such as task fixation (ie, repeatedly attempting futile SGA techniques). Unfamiliarity with invasive airway access techniques is a clear barrier to effective CICO crisis management.[9] The Difficult Airway Society guidelines recommend the scalpel technique as the first-line approach to CICO rescue given its high success rate and the ability to standardize and simplify training.[46] This approach, however, is subject to debate by others who contend that both needle and scalpel techniques are compatible with optimization of human factors in emergency airway management.[28,37] Regardless of the specific approach chosen, an individual's technical competency and familiarity with the invasive airway access technique are requisite for the successful management of a CICO emergency. To that end, simulation training using manikins, cadavers, or wet laboratory facilities is a practical method to educate and train anesthesiologists in the technical and nontechnical skills for airway management.[49] Trainees also can gain experience obtaining tracheal access with a catheter in live patients during elective procedures, such as translaryngeal blocks for awake flexible scope intubation.[50] Performing the procedure correctly to secure invasive airway access is among the last steps in a series of important decisions in a CICO emergency. Judgment errors and delaying the decision to obtain invasive airway access are significant contributors to morbidity and mortality in CICO scenarios.[6,7] During an emergency, activation of rehearsed responses from simulation training and the use of cognitive aids can mitigate the unproductive effects of stress on human behavior.[4,8]

Effective response in a high-acuity CICO scenario requires good teamwork, including effective communication, leadership, team coordination, and a shared understanding of roles.[39] Use of clear language and explicit declarations of a CICO emergency improves teamwork by creating a shared mental model and priming the team for an emergency surgical airway.[51] Help for additional airway expertise should be summoned early, ideally before the emergency invasive airway access pathway is encountered.[1,2,39] Clinicians called to help with airway management require clear instructions on what is expected of them. If possible, the team leader should remain hands-free to mitigate the risk of cognitive overload and to maintain situational awareness.[39] The team leader should carefully designate specific tasks, such as obtaining additional equipment and delegating further airway attempts to qualified team members.

The use of cognitive aids, such as the Vortex approach, can be an effective tool that is easily recalled by stressed clinicians and teams during difficult airway management.[4,47] This cognitive aid utilizes a visual aid in the shape of a funnel or vortex (**Fig. 3**) with an outer green zone that represents adequate alveolar oxygenation. Attempts to enter the green zone are made using the 3 lifelines or nonsurgical airway techniques: facemask ventilation, SGA, and tracheal intubation. If adequate alveolar oxygenation is not achieved despite best efforts at each of these lifelines, airway management proceeds down the vortex and requires emergency invasive surgical airway access (CICO rescue). Although the evidence base for this approach is limited, it has been developed with an emphasis on crisis management principles and human factors, offering conceptual advantages over traditional algorithmic approaches based on decision trees.

At an organizational level, a standardized difficult airway management strategy should be formulated by taking into account the specific needs, preferences, and skills of the clinicians involved in airway management. A portable storage unit containing standardized equipment for difficult airway management should be readily available to airway practitioners, who should be familiar with the location and storage of this equipment.[1] Specifically assembled and labeled CICO kits can be effective in improving the response to CICO emergencies.[28] Training for difficult airway

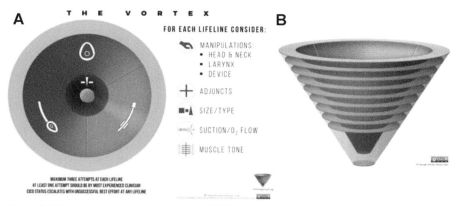

Fig. 3. (A) The Vortex implementation tool. (B) Lateral aspect of the Vortex in 3 dimensions, demonstrating the funnel concept. (*From* Chrimes N. The Vortex: a universal 'high-acuity implementation tool' for emergency airway management, *Br J Anaesth* 117:i20-i27, 2016; with permission.)

management should be provisioned to multidisciplinary teams at regular intervals through simulation-based training.[21] Although the available literature provides compelling evidence on the effectiveness of simulation-based training for invasive airway access,[52] there is limited evidence on how much and how often such training should be provided. Based on manikin studies, trainees are recommended to undergo at least 5 attempts at invasive airway access to become proficient in the technique.[53] Skills learned from simulation training in airway management can be retained for up to a year but skill fade can become apparent at approximately 6 months.[54] Training clinicians in both technical skills and nontechnical skills (eg, teamwork, communication, and situational awareness) is an important organizational component of human factors optimization in emergency airway management. Additional systemic efforts to improve difficult airway management should include adoption and implementation of best practice guidelines, use of preprocedural checklists and cognitive aids, collection of quality assurance data, and reporting of adverse events to registries.[8]

Clinics Care Points

- The anesthesiologist should always have a carefully planned strategy for airway management prior to the induction of anesthesia based on a comprehensive examination of the airway.

- Rescue of a CICO scenario should focus on emergency invasive airway access rather than relying on pharmacological intervention and awakening of the patient.

- It is important to have a standardized approach to invasive airway access at the local level with readily available equipment, consistent training, and skill maintenance programs.

- The "laryngeal handshake" technique is recommended over conventional palpation to improve the identification of the midline of the neck and CTM.

- A patent upper airway is required when using transtracheal jet ventilation in order to avoid barotrauma.

- Training for a response to the failed airway should include consideration of human factors at the individual, team, and organizational level.

DISCLOSURE

Dr C.A Hagberg has received funding for clinical research from Ambu, Karl Storz Endoscopy and Vyaire Medical. The other authors have no disclosures.

REFERENCES

1. Apfelbaum JL, Hagberg CA, Caplan RA, et al. Practice guidelines for management of the difficult airway an updated report by the American Society of Anesthesiologists Task Force on Management of the Difficult Airway. Anesthesiology 2013;118(2):251–70.
2. Frerk C, Mitchell VS, McNarry AF, et al. Difficult Airway Society 2015 guidelines for management of unanticipated difficult intubation in adults. Br J Anaesth 2015; 115(6):827–48.
3. Law JA, Broemling N, Cooper RM, et al. The difficult airway with recommendations for management–part 1–difficult tracheal intubation encountered in an unconscious/induced patient. Can J Anaesth 2013;60(11):1089–118.
4. Chrimes N. The Vortex: a universal "high-acuity implementation tool" for emergency airway management. Br J Anaesth 2016;117(Suppl 1):i20–7.
5. Cook TM, MacDougall-Davis SR. Complications and failure of airway management. Br J Anaesth 2012;109(Suppl 1):i68–85.
6. Cook TM, Woodall N, Frerk C. Fourth National Audit Project. Major complications of airway management in the UK: results of the Fourth National Audit Project of the Royal College of Anaesthetists and the Difficult Airway Society. Part 1: anaesthesia. Br J Anaesth 2011;106(5):617–31.
7. Joffe AM, Aziz MF, Posner KL, et al. Management of difficult tracheal IntubationA closed claims analysis. Anesthesiology 2019;131(4):818–29.
8. Watterson L, Rehak A, Heard A, et al. Transition from supraglottic to infraglottic rescue in the "can't intubate can't oxygenate"(CICO) scenario. 2014. Available at: https://researchmgt.monash.edu/ws/files/29924822/28568662_oa.pdf. Accessed April 29, 2020.
9. Greenland KB, Acott C, Segal R, et al. Emergency surgical airway in life-threatening acute airway emergencies–why are we so reluctant to do it? Anaesth Intensive Care 2011;39(4):578–84.
10. Gaba DM, Fish KJ, Howard SK, et al. Crisis management in anesthesiology E-Book. Philadelphia: Elsevier Health Sciences; 2014.
11. Crawley SM, Dalton AJ. Predicting the difficult airway. BJA Education 2015;15(5): 253–8.
12. Artime CA, Roy S, Hagberg CA. The difficult airway. Otolaryngol Clin North Am 2019;52(6):1115–25.
13. Kristensen MS, Teoh WH, Rudolph SS. Ultrasonographic identification of the cricothyroid membrane: best evidence, techniques, and clinical impact. Br J Anaesth 2016;117(Suppl 1):i39–48.
14. Naguib M, Brewer L, LaPierre C, et al. The Myth of rescue reversal in "can't intubate, can't ventilate" scenarios. Anesth Analg 2016;123(1):82–92.
15. Paton L, Gupta S, Blacoe D. Successful use of sugammadex in a "can"t ventilate' scenario. Anaesthesia 2013;68(8):861–4.
16. Lee C, Jahr JS, Candiotti K, et al. Reversal of profound rocuronium NMB with sugammadex is faster than recovery from succinylcholine. Anesthesiology 2007; 107:A988.

17. Bisschops MMA, Holleman C, Huitink JM. Can sugammadex save a patient in a simulated "cannot intubate, cannot ventilate" situation? Anaesthesia 2010;65(9): 936–41.
18. McGuire B, Dalton AJ. Sugammadex, airway obstruction, and drifting across the ethical divide: a personal account. Anaesthesia 2016;71(5):487–92.
19. Lockey D, Crewdson K, Weaver A, et al. Observational study of the success rates of intubation and failed intubation airway rescue techniques in 7256 attempted intubations of trauma patients by pre-hospital physicians. Br J Anaesth 2014; 113(2):220–5. Available at: https://www.ncbi.nlm.nih.gov/pubmed/25038154.
20. Baker PA, Weller JM, Greenland KB, et al. Education in airway management. Anaesthesia 2011;66(Suppl 2):101–11.
21. Kristensen MS, Teoh WHL, Baker PA. Percutaneous emergency airway access; prevention, preparation, technique and training. Br J Anaesth 2015;114(3): 357–61.
22. Cattano D, Cavallone L. Percutaneous dilational cricothyrotomy and tracheostomy. In: Hagberg CA, editor. Benumof and Hagberg's airway management. 3rd edition. Philadelphia: Elsevier Inc; 2012. p. 613–39.
23. Levitan RM. Tips and Tricks for Performing a Cricothyrotomy. ACEP Now 2014; 33(2). Available at: https://www.acepnow.com/article/tips-tricks-performing-cricothyrotomy/. Accessed October 8, 2020.
24. Hiller KN, Karni RJ, Cai C, et al. Comparing success rates of anesthesia providers versus trauma surgeons in their use of palpation to identify the cricothyroid membrane in female subjects: a prospective observational study. Can J Anaesth 2016; 63(7):807–17.
25. Siddiqui N, Yu E, Boulis S, et al. Ultrasound is superior to palpation in identifying the cricothyroid membrane in subjects with poorly defined neck landmarks: a randomized clinical trial. Anesthesiology 2018;129(6):1132–9.
26. You-Ten KE, Wong DT, Ye XY, et al. Practice of ultrasound-guided palpation of neck landmarks improves accuracy of external palpation of the cricothyroid membrane. Anesth Analg 2018;127(6):1377–82.
27. Langvad S, Hyldmo PK, Nakstad AR, et al. Emergency cricothyrotomy–a systematic review. Scand J Trauma Resusc Emerg Med 2013;21(1):43.
28. Booth AWG, Vidhani K. Human factors can't intubate can't oxygenate (CICO) bundle is more important than needle versus scalpel debate. Br J Anaesth 2017;118(3):466–8.
29. Price TM, McCoy EP. Emergency front of neck access in airway management. BJA Education 2019;19(8):246–53.
30. Scrase I, Woollard M. Needle vs surgical cricothyroidotomy: a short cut to effective ventilation. Anaesthesia 2006;61(10):962–74.
31. DeVore EK, Redmann A, Howell R, et al. Best practices for emergency surgical airway: a systematic review. Laryngoscope Investig Otolaryngol 2019;4(6):602–8.
32. Mace SE, Khan N. Needle cricothyrotomy. Emerg Med Clin North Am 2008;26(4): 1085–101, xi.
33. Duggan LV, Ballantyne Scott B, Law JA, et al. Transtracheal jet ventilation in the 'can't intubate can't oxygenate' emergency: a systematic review. Br J Anaesth 2016;117(Suppl 1):i28–38.
34. Melker JS, Gabrielli A. Melker cricothyrotomy kit: an alternative to the surgical technique. Ann Otol Rhinol Laryngol 2005;114(7):525–8.
35. Heard AMB, Green RJ, Eakins P. The formulation and introduction of a "can't intubate, can't ventilate" algorithm into clinical practice. Anaesthesia 2009;64(6): 601–8.

36. Eisenburger P, Laczika K, List M, et al. Comparison of conventional surgical versus seldinger technique emergency cricothyrotomy performed by inexperienced clinicians. Anesthesiology 2000;92(3):687–90.
37. Heard A, Dinsmore J, Douglas S, et al. Plan D: cannula first, or scalpel only? Br J Anaesth 2016;117(4):533–5.
38. Engels PT, Bagshaw SM, Meier M, et al. Tracheostomy: from insertion to decannulation. Can J Surg 2009;52(5):427–33.
39. Higgs A, McGrath BA, Goddard C, et al. Guidelines for the management of tracheal intubation in critically ill adults. Br J Anaesth 2018;120(2):323–52.
40. Heffner JE. Tracheotomy application and timing. Clin Chest Med 2003;24(3): 389–98.
41. Warner MA, Smith HM, Zielinski MD. Impaired ventilation and oxygenation after emergency cricothyrotomy: recommendations for the management of suboptimal invasive airway Access. A A Case Rep 2016;7(10):212–4.
42. Talving P, DuBose J, Inaba K, et al. Conversion of emergent cricothyrotomy to tracheotomy in trauma patients. Arch Surg 2010;145(1):87–91.
43. Feinleib J, Foley L, Mark L. What we all should know about our patient's airway. Anesthesiol Clin 2015;33(2):397–413.
44. Gazoni FM, Amato PE, Malik ZM, et al. The impact of perioperative catastrophes on anesthesiologists: results of a national survey. Anesth Analg 2012;114(3): 596–603.
45. Fanning RM, Gaba DM. Debriefing. Crisis management in anesthesiology. 2nd edition. Philadelphia: Elsevier Saunders; 2015. p. 65–78.
46. Moneypenny MJ. When are "human factors" not "human factors" in can't intubate can't oxygenate scenarios? When they are "human" factors. Br J Anaesth 2017; 118(3):469.
47. The Vortex Approach. The Vortex Approach. Available at: http://vortexapproach. org. Accessed April 30, 2020.
48. LeBlanc VR. The effects of acute stress on performance: implications for health professions education. Acad Med 2009;84(10 Suppl):S25–33.
49. Komasawa N, Berg BW. Simulation-based Airway Management Training for Anesthesiologists - A brief review of its essential role in skills training for clinical competency. J Educ Perioper Med 2017;19(4):E612.
50. Timmermann A, Chrimes N, Hagberg CA. Need to consider human factors when determining first-line technique for emergency front-of-neck access. Br J Anaesth 2016;117(1):5–7.
51. Chrimes N, Cook TM. Critical airways, critical language. Br J Anaesth 2017; 119(5):1072.
52. Yang D, Wei Y-K, Xue F-S, et al. Simulation-based airway management training: application and looking forward. J Anesth 2016;30(2):284–9.
53. Shetty K, Nayyar V, Stachowski E, et al. Training for cricothyroidotomy. Anaesth Intensive Care 2013;41(5):623–30.
54. Hubert V, Duwat A, Deransy R, et al. Effect of simulation training on compliance with difficult airway management algorithms, technical ability, and skills retention for emergency cricothyrotomy. Anesthesiology 2014;120(4):999–1008.

The Septic Patient

Arpit Patel, MD, Mark E. Nunnally, MD*

KEYWORDS

- Source control • Resuscitation • Stroke volume variation • Cardiomyopathy
- Driving pressure

KEY POINTS

- Anesthesiologists need a careful plan of induction that includes being wary of ileus, aspiration, and cardiovascular collapse.
- The therapeutic focus in sepsis should be on achieving source control and initiation of early broad-spectrum antibiotics.
- Dynamic fluid responsiveness might be a way to minimize over-resuscitation.
- Assessment of circulatory failure involves both right ventricular function and left ventricular function.
- Evaluating driving pressure mechanics can aid in optimizing positive end-expiratory pressure.

INTRODUCTION

Sepsis is a leading cause of death worldwide, leading to approximately 49,000,000 cases and 11,000,000 deaths per year[1]—312,000 deaths per year in the United States.[2] It affects anyone, young or old, and is the final common pathway for some fatal diseases, such as advanced cancer. Independent of mortality, sepsis is striking in the toll it takes on survivors, many of whom survive with cognitive and functional decline and some of whom continue to need advanced therapies. Contrasting these outcomes with the observation that early therapies improve outcomes, sepsis is one of the great therapeutic opportunities in acute care medicine.

A subset of sepsis patients presents with surgical pathology. For these patients, essential source control requires emergent operation. Because of the urgency of timely therapy, it is important to emphasize that priority is on timely surgery rather than medical stabilization. Because anesthesiologists are experts at resuscitation, titration, and monitoring, they are uniquely suited to help care for sepsis patients and their role is crucial to altering the trajectory of life-threatening illness. Surgical sepsis is an emergency.

Department of Anesthesiology, Perioperative Care and Pain Medicine, NYU Langone Health, NYU Langone Medical Center, 550 1st Avenue, New York, NY 10016, USA
* Corresponding author.
E-mail address: Mark.Nunnally@nyulangone.org

Anesthesiology Clin 38 (2020) 889–899
https://doi.org/10.1016/j.anclin.2020.08.004
1932-2275/20/© 2020 Elsevier Inc. All rights reserved.

Anesthesiologists must be prepared to facilitate this emergent care and need to understand the considerations sepsis has for the management of an anesthetic and postoperative care.

SOURCE CONTROL

Anesthesiologists need to adapt to uncertain and suboptimal physiologic conditions because early source control for septic patients should be considered an emergency. Source control and early antibiotics are paramount in the management of the septic patient. Delay in any of these treatments leads to a further dysregulated host response to infection. Each hour in delay of early broad-spectrum antibiotics adds approximately a 7% increase in mortality over the first 6 hours.[3] Early strategy should focus on source control, resuscitation with intravenous (IV) fluids, broad-spectrum antibiotics, maintaining oxygenation and ventilation, and restoration of hemodynamics. Source control should be delayed only when clinically appropriate. Excessive diagnostic testing and consultation prior to achievement of source control leads to an increase in adverse events.

INDUCTION OF THE CRITICALLY ILL

Induction of anesthesia in the critically ill patient requires careful evaluation of the neurologic, respiratory, cardiovascular, and gastrointestinal systems. Sepsis patients have high adrenergic tone and induction agents should be dosed to minimize hemodynamic effects, in particular hypotension. It also should be noted that ileus is often under-recognized in sepsis and these patients should be considered to have full stomachs on induction. Nonabdominal sources of sepsis still are at risk from aspiration.

Choice of induction agent involves an individualized approach and standard doses should be avoided. Commonly used medications include opioids, benzodiazepines, lidocaine, propofol, etomidate, and ketamine along with a neuromuscular blockers. Laryngoscopy can lead to hemodynamic instability, including tachycardia and hypertension, which can in turn increase myocardial demand. In the postinduction/intubation period, there often is an attenuation of sympathetic tone followed by hypotension. It, therefore, is important to have adequate IV access and readily available vasopressors and IV fluids.

The choice of etomidate as an induction agent may help prevent hemodynamic depression, but its value is unsubstantiated in trials of critically ill patients. Subgroups with sepsis from these trials fared worse, with a tendency toward increased mortality with etomidate.[4] This finding may be due to the tendency of etomidate to suppress the adrenal axis, leading to increased hemodynamic instability in septic patients.

MONITORING

Monitoring of patients in the perioperative period is important for titration of resuscitation in sepsis. Arterial lines provide valuable information in real time and often are indicated when actively resuscitating a septic patient, to allow for improved titration of anesthetics and vasopressors and to trend arterial blood gases. Furthermore, arterial line waveform interpretations, such as pulse pressure variation (PPV) and stroke volume variation (SVV), are dynamic and, therefore, may be the most reliable measures of fluid responsiveness.

Optimizing preload and correcting hypovolemia in order to maximize cardiac output early can help to improve outcome and minimize side effects from vasopressor use. Up to 50% of patients no longer may be volume responsive after initial resuscitation.[5]

It is likely volume requirements shift in most resuscitations from intravascular deficit to surplus. Targeted monitoring strategies enable a timely shift in the goals of therapy. Retrospective data from an acute respiratory distress syndrome (ARDS) cohort and data from a vasopressin trial suggest an association with positive cumulative fluid balance and complications, including, mortality, and length of intensive care unit (ICU) stay.[6]

PULSE PRESSURE VARIATION AND STROKE VOLUME VARIATION

SVV and PVV are real-time dynamic tests of the effects of changes to ventricular filling. The principle is based on changes in intrathoracic pressure during positive pressure ventilation. Mechanical ventilation causes a transient increase in left ventricular (LV) preload, followed by a decrease in right ventricular (RV) preload and an increase in RV afterload translating to an increase and then a decrease in LV filling and ejection. This phenomenon is magnified on the steeper portions of the Frank-Starling curve.[7] A variation of 12% to 13% is highly predictive of volume responsiveness,[7] meaning that clinicians can, if they feel the circulation is inadequate, administer fluids. Using PPV as a second check on volume decisions aids in resuscitation tied to physiologic endpoints.

New commercial products have been developed based on the principles of SVV as a marker for resuscitation responsiveness (**Fig. 1**). These products have of the advantage of being noninvasive.[8] Ultimately, they should serve as an adjunct tool and not a replacement for clinical judgment. SVV assessment has its own limitations. Arrhythmias, spontaneous ventilation, and importantly low-tidal-volume ventilation cause misinterpretation of SVV.[9] Importantly, tidal volumes ideally should be 8 mL/kg to 10 mL/kg ideal body weight to predict fluid responsiveness, but, when not being measured, many sepsis patients should be ventilated with lower volumes.[9]

Similar to SVV, analysis of plethysmograph waveforms may be useful in predicting fluid responsiveness.[10,11] The pulse oximeter waveform can be viewed as an extension of the peripheral arterial waveform, and the differences in peak and trough of

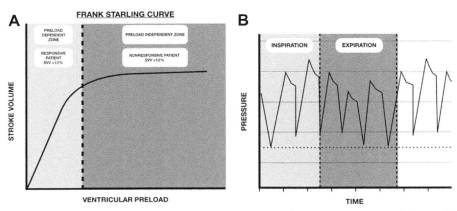

Fig. 1. (A) SVV and the Frank-Starling curve. In the zone of the ascending limb of the Frank-Starling curve, an SVV greater than 12% indicates volume responsiveness. The shallow part of the curve (SVV <12%) indicates a nonresponder to volume. (B) This graph shows the correlation of the rising intrathoracic pressure, which in turn causes a decrease RV preload during inspiration. LV preload is sequentially affected after a few heart beats, which is reflected during the expiratory cycle.

the plethysmograph during the respiratory cycle align well to arterial measurements.[12] When faced with multiple tasks, and unable to efficiently place an arterial line in time, utilizing the plethysmograph waveform as an adjunct provides valuable data.

Central venous monitoring, although predictive of right atrial pressure, is unreliable as a dynamic marker of fluid responsiveness and as a marker of resuscitation. It traditionally has been used in both the operating room and ICU to help guide fluid management.[13] Acute changes in central venous pressure (CVP) and its trend overtime can produce clinically valuable data, but over-reliance on CVP alone can be misleading.

In most clinical settings, clinicians no longer use pulmonary artery catheter routinely. They provide data regarding cardiac filling pressures, but these are susceptible to variability in clinicians' interpretations. Trials in patients with ARDS or shock suggest no mortality benefit with pulmonary artery catheter–guided decision making.[14,15] Dynamic markers of resuscitation, including SVV and plethysmography analysis, are the preferred clinical tools for volume management.

TISSUE OXYGENATION/PERFUSION

One salient goal of care for patients in septic shock is maintaining adequate oxygenation and tissue perfusion. **Table 1** lists clinical markers useful in assessing perfusion. Mentation may be used as a clinical index prior to induction but may be directly depressed by sepsis. Elevated serum lactate is a marker of tissue hypoperfusion, and frequent assessment of lactate levels is endorsed by the Surviving Sepsis Campaign.[16] Assessment of lactate as frequently as every 2 hours to 4 hours may help with resuscitation and is a predictor of mortality.[17–21] Early lactate clearance in shock is an independent predictor for survival.[20] Lactate production and delayed clearance, however, may be due to multiple factors and not linked directly to fluid resuscitation alone. The activation of the adrenergic sympathetic system and β_1-agonists raise lactate levels.[16]

Although having a quantitative laboratory measurement would be ideal, no 1 metric for tissue oxygenation is completely reliable. Physical examination and serial capillary refill examinations as endpoints of resuscitation seem to perform comparably with a lactate clearance strategy, measured by all-cause 90-day mortality.[22] Constant vigilance and re-evaluation of clinical trends are the best approaches to the complex problem of septic shock management.

FLUID RESUSCITATION

Recommended IV fluid bolusing, administered at 30 mL/kg over the first 3 hours, is a reasonable guideline but should be adjusted to clinical circumstances. Clinicians should continue fluid resuscitation if hemodynamics improve with ongoing fluid

Table 1	
Perfusion indicators that can be helpful in assessing a patient with sepsis	
Clinical Indices of Perfusion	**Laboratory Indices of Prefusion**
• MAP	• Blood lactate
• Mentation	• Mixed venous oxygen saturation
• Urine output	• Arterial pH, BE, HCO_3
• Cool extremities	
• Capillary refill	
• Abdominal ischemia/ileus	

Abbreviations: BE, base excess; HCO_3, bicarbonate.

challenges.[16] As a general rule, IV fluids should be administered more liberally in the active resuscitative phase of shock. With shock resolution, management should be more conservative, weighing hazards against benefits.

IV crystalloids are to be first line in critically ill patients. Iatrogenic hyperchloremia contributes to kidney injury. Trials comparing balanced crystalloids (lactated Ringer solution and Plasma-Lyte 148 [Baxter International, Deerfield, IL]) with 0.9% normal saline in critically ill patients suggest mortality and acute kidney injury are reduced using a balanced solution.[23] Concerns of hyperkalemia when giving Ringer solution to critically ill patients with renal injury often are exaggerated.[24]

Albumin has been studied extensively as a resuscitative fluid in patients with sepsis. With a longer intravascular half-life than crystalloids, it potentially can decrease interstitial fluid accumulation. Albumin is more expensive. There appears to be no difference in all-cause mortality between albumin and saline; however, traumatic brain injury patients may fare worse with albumin administration.[25] Albumin resuscitation in sepsis did not influence mortality in a trial design, but its use has been associated with lower Sequential Organ Failure Assessment (SOFA) scores and vasopressor doses.[26] Albumin may confer an advantage when patients require substantial amounts of fluid repletion.[16] A strategy that employs using albumin along with crystalloid may be beneficial when patients are suffering from side effects of over-resuscitation, such as pulmonary and bowel edema.

Starches have been extensively used in the operating room and ICUs for volume expansion. Lower-molecular-weight preparations purportedly prevent acute kidney injury and coagulopathy. A meta-analysis of studies suggests, however, increased incidence of renal replacement therapy and a trend toward higher overall mortality compared with albumin or IV fluids.[16,27] Starches no longer are recommended in sepsis.

CARDIOMYOPATHY IN SEPSIS

Some patients with sepsis commonly develop cardiovascular abnormalities. Echocardiographic data indicate up to a 40% incidence of myocardial hypokinesis in patients with sepsis.[28] Initially, cardiac output is decreased in sepsis secondary to low intravascular volume. Early fluid resuscitation in combination with low systemic vascular resistance increases cardiac output. LV dilation leads to higher stroke volume, despite lower contractility. and is described in sepsis survivors.[29] The dilation of the LV may be a naturally occurring adaptive response.[29,30] Sepsis-induced cardiomyopathy appears to be different from cardiomyopathy without sepsis, because it typically is limited and reversible in 7 days to 10 days with supportive care.

RV failure likely is under-recognized in sepsis, and failure to understand how to optimize RV physiology can increase mortality. In the presence of decreased contractility and increased pulmonary vascular resistance, there may be insufficient filling of the RV, causing it to become the output-limiting chamber.[31] In a survey of septic shock patients, depressed RV function was a common finding in nonsurvivors.[32]

Currently, there are no further guidelines in treating sepsis-induced cardiomyopathy beyond usual care. There is no survival benefit in the early administration of dobutamine or other inotropes. Norepinephrine should remain as first-line therapy for initial hemodynamic instability.[30,33]

OPTIMAL PERFUSION PRESSURE AND PRESSORS

A mean arterial pressure (MAP) of 65 mm Hg generally is accepted as the perfusion pressure to maintain oxygen delivery to the vital organs. This MAP goal should not distract from the importance organ-specific blood flow. This differs in each patient, and patients with chronic hypertension may require higher perfusion pressures or prevent end organ damage. There is a tradeoff between perfusion pressure and adverse effects of vasopressors.[34] Central venous catheters provide a reliable and safe route for vasopressor administration, but line placement may lead to delays in treatment. Timely placement of large-bore peripheral access allows for rapid resuscitation and ability to administer peripheral vasopressors. Distal catheter placement and use for greater than 24 hours are major risk factors for tissue injury from vasopressor extravasation.[35] Less concentrated vasopressors might mitigate the risk.

Phenylephrine and ephedrine are the immediate vasopressors used by anesthesiologists that are available most commonly . These medications should be used cautiously as temporizing measures in patients with sepsis. First-line vasopressor therapy in sepsis includes the early use of norepinephrine for immediate restoration of hemodynamics.[16] Epinephrine or vasopressin should be considered sequentially, depending on the clinical scenario. The lactic acidosis directly produced by epinephrine likely is not of clinical significance.[36] Mesenteric ischemia is a commonly feared consequence of vasopressor use. No known vasopressor can mitigate against this risk. Natural vasopressin levels are reduced in the septic state, and addition of low-dose vasopressin can improve hemodynamics[16,37,38] (**Table 2**).

VENTILATORY STRATEGIES

Anesthesiologists can provide a valuable role titrating mechanical ventilation in the operating room. Mechanical ventilation of patients with the ARDS puts them at an increased risk of mortality.[39] The fundamental goals are the prevention of volutrauma and barotrauma and positive end-expiratory pressure (PEEP) optimization.

Low-tida- volume ventilation is strongly recommended in ARDS.[40] Use of lower tidal volume at 6 mL/kg of ideal body weight and limitation of plateau pressures between 25 mm Hg and 30 mm Hg are associated with an overall benefit in mortality reduction and ventilator-free days.[40] These parameters are now standards of care among patients in ARDS and there are data suggesting that the practice decreases lung inflammatory markers, progression to ARDS, and postoperative pulmonary complications.[39,40]

Optimization of PEEP by calculating driving pressure is a tool for anesthesiologists to use in the operating room. Driving pressure easily can be calculated using plateau pressure (PEEP). The driving pressure in an indirect measure of alveolar and lung compliance. If, by increasing PEEP, more lung volume is recruited, driving pressures

Table 2
Vasopressors used in sepsis

Drug	Dose	Receptor				
		α	$\beta1$	$\beta2$	Dopamine	Vasopressin
Norepinephrine (μg/min)	0.5–30	+ + + +	+ +	–	–	–
Epinephrine (μg/kg/min)	0.01–0.05	+	+ + +	+ +	–	–
	>0.05	+ + +	+ +	+ +	–	–
Vasopressin (units/min)	0.01–0.06	–	–	–	–	+ + +
Dopamine (μg/kg/min)	0.5–5	–	+	–	+ + + +	–
	5–10	+	+ +	–	+ + +	–
	10–20	+ + +	+ +	–	+	–
Phenylephrine μg/min	10–300	+ + +	–	–	–	–

decrease for the same size tidal volume, demonstrating improved respiratory system compliance. On the other hand, if PEEP is increased and driving pressure increases, it suggests alveolar over-distension. Further increases in PEEP are harmful to the lungs. A reanalysis of 9 major ARDS trials suggests that a decreased driving pressure independently favors mortality.[41] Clinicians should aim for a decreased change in pressure and driving pressure less than 15 cm H_2O^{40-43} (**Table 3**).

The use of higher PEEP comes with the risks of increased strain on the RV and increased intrathoracic pressure, which can limit preload. Caution should be exercised when employing a high PEEP strategy in patients who are inadequately volume resuscitated.

No specific mode of mechanical ventilation offers a mortality benefit when applying the principles of limiting volume and pressure. The volume control mode used in most operating room ventilators allows an accurate assessment of plateau pressures, but some operating room ventilators may not offer an inspiratory pause maneuver to measure plateau pressure. Pressure control modes may be beneficial by delivering a decelerating flow pattern, which is analogous to a physiologic inspiration. Hybrid modes now are available on most new anesthesia machines, purportedly offering the benefit of a volume target with a pressure limit. It is important for anyone providing ventilator management in the operating room to be comfortable with all modes of ventilation.

METABOLIC ACIDOSIS AND USE OF SODIUM BICARBONATE

Metabolic acidosis frequently is encountered in sepsis. Severe acidosis may result in vasodilation, further compounding hypotension in sepsis. Currently, routine use of sodium bicarbonate in the presence of a pH higher than 7.15 is not recommended.[16,44] Sodium bicarbonate does not reverse the lactic acidosis associated with hypoperfusion. Risks associated with bolus or infusion of sodium bicarbonate include worsening respiratory acidosis, hypocalcemia, hypernatremia, and intravascular volume overload. Immediate hemodynamic benefits of sodium bicarbonate bolus likely are from an intravascular osmolar load and increased preload. Benefits of bicarbonate infusion may be to decrease the need for renal replacement therapy in patients with an acute kidney injury.[45]

STEROIDS/VITAMIN C/THIAMINE

Sepsis alters mineralocorticoid and glucocorticoid secretion. Despite endocrine dysregulation, administration of steroids remains a clinically unsettled practice. Benefits

Table 3
Review of data from Amato and colleagues[41] shows the correlation of driving pressure and mortality in the context of rising airway pressures.

Plateau Pressure	Positive End-Expiratory Pressure	Driving Pressure	Mortality
↑	Same	↑	↑
↑	↑	Same	Same
Same	↑	↓	↓

Higher plateau pressures or higher positive end-expiratory pressure did not affect mortality if driving pressure remained unchanged.

From Amato MB, Meade MO, Slutsky AS. Driving pressure and survival in the acute respiratory distress syndrome. The New England journal of medicine. 2015 372(8):747-55.; with permission.

include data suggesting improvement in SOFA scores and reduced vasoconstrictor use.[46–48] Use may lead, however, to hypernatremia, hyperglycemia, and risks of further immune compromise.[46] Early steroid administration in vasopressor resistant shock is associated with reversal of shock, but data have been equivocal with respect to mortality.[49]

Recent data have renewed interest in administration of vitamin C and thiamine in sepsis. Proposed mechanisms for vitamin C include a role in maintenance of the endothelium and decreasing capillary leak.[50–52] Thiamine may play an integral role in metabolic pathways, because repletion can increase lactate clearance in some patients.[53] Each therapy is awaiting further validation from randomized controlled trials. If proved, they may be an attractive option with relatively low cost and toxicity profile.

HYPERGLYCEMIA

Blood glucose regulation frequently is altered in sepsis. Frequently, hyperglycemia is a part of the stress response. Titration of insulin to a blood glucose goal less than 180 mg/dL is a current standard of practice based on minimizing harms from hyperglycemia and risks from intensive insulin therapy.[54,55] Targeting blood glucose levels below 120 mg/dL is not recommended as hypoglycemia and mortality seem to increase at this level of intensity. Challenges in IV insulin administration include drug incompatibly with other IV medications and frequent monitoring needs.[54,55]

TRANSPORT TO INTENSIVE CARE UNIT

Transportation of critically ill patients to and from the operating room to the ICU requires an organized and methodical approach. For patients in ARDS requiring high ventilatory support, the use of a travel ventilator instead of an inflatable bag prevents derecruitment and worsening oxygenation. Emergency resuscitation medications, including IV fluids, should be readily available. Proper sedation prevents recall. Surgical and anesthesia teams should discuss the case with the ICU nurse and provider team to ensure consensus thinking and continuity of care.

SUMMARY

The evolution of sepsis care reflects a sequence of discarded theories, and that sequence describes the evolution of our understanding that this is not a simple process based on a toxin or a cytokine. Rather, the complex, whole-body response to infection suggests a cellular lesion that has implications for the coordination of tissues and organs.[56] Attempts to block specific components of the inflammatory cascade or to blunt it broadly have been unsuccessful.[57] What has persisted is a focus on source control, timely targeted resuscitation, and rapid and appropriate treatment with antibiotics. An anesthesiologist facilitates these interventions for patients requiring operative and postoperative care. Although research efforts continue to seek a method to reverse the physiologic derangements in sepsis, for now, attention to detail and timely response are what matter most.

DISCLOSURE

No financial disclosures.

REFERENCES

1. Rudd KE, Johnson SC, Agesa KM, et al. Global, regional, and national sepsis incidence and mortality, 1990-2017: analysis for the global burden of disease study. Lancet 2020;395:200–11.
2. Paoli C, Reynolds M, Sinha M, et al. Epidemiology and costs of sepsis in the United States-an analysis based on timing if diagnosis and severity level. Crit Care Med 2018;46:1889–97.
3. Kumar A, Roberts D, Wood KE, et al. Duration of hypotension before initiation of effective antimicrobial therapy is the critical determinant of survival in human septic shock. Crit Care Med 2006;34:1589–96.
4. Jabre P, Combes X, Lapostolle F, et al. Etomidate versus ketamine for rapid sequence intubation in acutely ill patients: a multicenter randomized controlled trial. Lancet 2009;374(9686):293–300.
5. Marik PE, Cavallazzi R, Vasu T, et al. Dynamic changes in arterial waveform derived variables and fluid responsiveness in mechanically ventilated patients. A systematic review of the literature. Crit Care Med 2009;37:2642–7.
6. Rosenberg AL, Dechert RE, Park PK, et al. Review of a large clinical series: association of cumulative fluid balance on outcome in acute lung injury: a retrospective review of the ARDSnet tidal volume study cohort. J Intensive Care Med 2009; 24:35–46.
7. Marik PE, Monnet X, Teboul JL. Hemodynamic parameters to guide fluid therapy. Ann Intensive Care 2011;1:1.
8. Sumiyoshi M, Maeda T, Miyazaki E, et al. Accuracy of the Clear- SightTM system in patients undergoing abdominal aortic aneurysm surgery. J Anesth 2019;33:364–71.
9. Reuter DA, Bayerlein J, Goepfert MSG, et al. Influence of tidal volume on left ventricular stroke volume variation measured by pulse contour analysis in mechanically ventilated patients. Intensive Care Med 2003;29(3):476–80.
10. Cannesson M, Besnard C, Durand PG, et al. Relation between respiratory variations in pulse oximetry plethysmographic waveform amplitude and arterial pulse pressure in ventilated patients. Crit Care 2005;9:R562–8.
11. Cannesson M, Musard H, Desebbe O, et al. The ability of stroke volume variations obtained with Vigileo/FloTrac system to monitor fluid responsiveness in mechanically ventilated patients. Anesth Analg 2009;108:513–7.
12. Feissel M, Teboul JL, Merlani P, et al. Plethysmographic dynamic indices predict fluid responsiveness in septic ventilated patients. Intensive Care Med 2007;33:993–9.
13. Kastrup M, Markewitz A, Spies C, et al. Current practice of hemodynamic monitoring and vasopressor and inotropic therapy in post-operative cardiac surgery patients in Germany: results from a postal survey. Acta Anaesthesiol Scand 2007;51:347–58.
14. Wheeler AP, Bernard GR, Thompson BT, et al. Pulmonary artery versus central venous catheter to guide treatment of acute lung injury. N Engl J Med 2006; 354(21):2213–24.
15. Harvey S, Harrison DA, Singer M, et al. Assessment of the clinical effectiveness of pulmonary artery catheters in management of patients in intensive care (PAC-Man): a randomized controlled trial. Lancet 2005;366(9484):472–7.
16. Rhodes A, Evans LE, Alhazzani W, et al. Surviving sepsis campaign: international guidelines for management of sepsis and septic shock: 2016. Intensive Care Med 2017;43(3):304–77.
17. Marik PE, Bellomo R, Demla V. Lactate clearance as a target of therapy in sepsis: a flawed paradigm. OA Crit Care 2013;1(1):3.

18. Regnier MA, Raux M, Le MY, et al. Prognostic significance of blood lactate and lactate clearance in trauma patients. Anesthesiology 2012;117(6):1276–88.
19. Manikis P, Jankowski S, Zhang H, et al. Correlation of serial blood lactate levels to organ failure and mortality after trauma. Am J Emerg Med 1995;13(6):619–22.
20. Jansen TC, van Bommel J, Schoonderbeek FJ, et al. Early lactate-guided therapy in intensive care unit patients: a multicenter, open-label, randomized controlled trial. Am J Respir Crit Care Med 2010;182(6):752–61.
21. Mikkelsen ME, Miltiades AN, Gaieski, et al. Serum lactate is associated with mortality in severe sepsis independent of organ failure and shock. Crit Care Med 2009;37(5):1670–7.
22. Hernández G, Ospina-Tascón GA, Petri Damiani L, et al. Effect of a resuscitation strategy targeting peripheral perfusion status vs serum lactate levels on 28-day mortality among patients with septic shock: the ANDROMEDA-SHOCK randomized clinical trial. JAMA 2019;321(7):654–64.
23. Semler MW, Self WH, Wanderer JP, et al. Balanced crystalloids versus saline in critically ill adults. N Engl J Med 2018;378(9):829–39.
24. Nunnally ME, Patel A. Sepsis-What's new in 2019? Curr Opin Anesthesiol 2019; 32(2):163–8.
25. Finfer S, Bellomo R, Boyce N, et al. A comparison of albumin and saline for fluid resuscitation in the intensive care unit". N Engl J Med 2004;350(22):2247–56.
26. Caironi P, Tognoni G, Masson S, et al. Albumin replacement in patients with severe sepsis or septic shock. N Engl J Med 2014;370(15):1412–21.
27. Haase N, Perner A, Hennings LI, et al. Hydroxyethyl starch 130/0.38-0.45 versus crystalloid or albumin in patients with sepsis: systematic review with meta-analysis and trial sequential analysis. BMJ 2013;346:f839.
28. Vieillard-Baron A, Caille V, Charron C, et al. Actual incidence of global left ventricular hypokinesia in adult septic shock. Crit Care Med 2008;36(6):1701–6.
29. Zanotti Cavazzoni SL, Guglielmi M, Parrillo JE, et al. Ventricular dilation is associated with improved cardiovascular performance and survival in sepsis. Chest 2010;138:848–55.
30. Sato R, Nasu M. A review of sepsis-induced cardiomyopathy. J Intensive Care 2015;3(1):48.
31. Chan CM, Klinger JR. The right ventricle in sepsis. Clin Chest Med 2008;29(4):661–76.
32. Furian T, Aguiar C, Prado K, et al. Ventricular dysfunction and dilation in severe sepsis and septic shock: relation to endothelial function and mortality. J Crit Care 2012;27(3):319.e9.
33. Gattinoni L, Brazzi L, Pelosi P, et al. A trial of goal- oriented hemodynamic therapy in critically ill patients. ScvO2 Collaborative Group. N Engl J Med 1995;333(16): 1025–32.
34. De Backer D, Creteur J, Silva E, et al. Effects of dopamine, norepinephrine, and epinephrine on the splanchnic circulation in septic shock: which is best? Crit Care Med 2003;31(6):1659–67.
35. Lewis Tyler, Merchan C, Altshuler D, et al. Safety of the peripheral administration of vasopressor agents. J Intensive Care Med 2019;34(1):26–33.
36. Myburgh JA, Higgins A, Jovanovska A, et al. A comparison of epinephrine and norepinephrine in critically ill patients. Intensive Care Med 2008;34(12):2226–34.
37. Patel BM, Chittock DR, Russell JA, et al. Beneficial effects of short-term vasopressin infusion during severe septic shock. Anesthesiology 2002;96(3):576–82.
38. Dunser MW, Mayr AJ, Ulmer H, et al. Arginine vasopressin in advanced vasodilatory shock: a prospective, randomized, controlled study. Circulation 2003; 107(18):2313–9.

39. Neto AS, Cardoso SO, Manetta JA, et al. Association between use of lung-protective ventilation with lower tidal volumes and clinical outcomes among patients without acute respiratory distress syndrome: a meta-analysis. JAMA 2012;308(16):1651–9.
40. Brower RG, Matthay MA, Morris A, et al. Ventilation with lower tidal volumes as compared with traditional tidal volumes for acute lung injury and the acute respiratory distress syndrome. N Engl J Med 2000;342(18):1301–8.
41. Amato MB, Meade MO, Slutsky AS. Driving pressure and survival in the acute respiratory distress syndrome. N Engl J Med 2015;372(8):747–55.
42. Futier E, Constantin JM, Paugam-Burtz C, et al. A trial of intraoperative low-tidal-volume ventilation in abdominal surgery. N Engl J Med 2013;369(5):428–37.
43. Bugedo G, Retamal J, Bruhn A. Driving pressure: a marker of severity, a safety limit, or a goal for mechanical ventilation? Crit Care 2017;21:199.
44. Mathieu D, Neviere R, Billard V, et al. Effects of bicarbonate therapy on hemodynamics and tissue oxygenation in patients with lactic acidosis: a prospective, controlled clinical study. Crit Care Med 1991;19(11):1352–6.
45. Jaber S, Paugam C, Futier E, et al. Sodium bicarbonate therapy for patients with severe metabolic acidemia in the intensive care unit (BICAR-ICU): a multicenter, open-label, randomized controlled, phase 3 trial. Lancet 2018;392(10141):31–40.
46. Rochwerg B, Oczkowski SJ, Siemieniuk RA, et al. Corticosteroids in sepsis: an updated systematic review and meta-analysis. Crit Care Med 2018;46:1411–20.
47. Annane D, Sebile V, Charpentier C, et al. Effect of treatment with low doses ofhydrocortisone and fludrocortisone on mortality in patients with septic shock. J Am Med Assoc 2002;288:862–71.
48. Sprung CL, Annane D, Keh D, et al. Hydrocortisone therapy for patients with septic shock. N Engl J Med 2008;358:111.
49. Gajic O, Ahmad S, Wilson M, et al. Outcomes of critical illness: what is meaningful? Curr Opin Crit Care 2018;24:394–400.
50. Zhou G, Kamenos G, Pendem S, et al. Ascorbate protects against vascular leakage in cecal ligation, and puncture induced septic peritonitis. Am J Physiol Regul Integr Comp Physiol 2012;302:R409–16.
51. Fowler AA, Syed AA, Knowlson S, et al. Phase 1 safety trial of intravenous ascorbic acid in patients with severe sepsis. J Transl Med 2014;12:32.
52. Tanaka H, Matsuda T, Miyagantani Y, et al. Reduction of resuscitation fluid volumes in severely burned patients using ascorbic acid administration; a randomized, prospective study. Arch Surg 2000;135:326–31.
53. Woolum J, Abner EL, Kelly A, et al. Effect of thiamine administration on lactate clearance and mortality in patients with septic shock. Crit Care Med 2018;46:1747–52.
54. Van den Berghe G, Wouters P, Weekers F, et al. Intensive insulin therapy in critically ill patients. N Engl J Med 2001;345(19):1359–67.
55. Van den Berghe G, Wilmer A, Hermans G, et al. Intensive insulin therapy in the medical ICU. N Engl J Med 2006;354(5):449–61.
56. Godin PJ, Buchman TG. Uncoupling of biological oscillators: a complementary hypothesis concerning the pathogenesis of multiple organ dysfunction syndrome. Crit Care Med 1996;24(7):1107–16.
57. Abraham E, Wunderink R, Silverman H, et al. Efficacy and safety of monoclonal antibody to human tumor necrosis factor alpha in patients with sepsis syndrome. A randomized, controlled double-blind, multicenter clinical trial. TNF-alpha Mab Sepsis Study Group. JAMA 1995;273(12):934–41.

Failures of the Oxygen Supply

Richard Botney, MD[a],*, Joseph F. Answine, MD[b,c,d,e,1],
Charles E. Cowles Jr, MD, MBA[f]

KEYWORDS

- Anesthesia • Oxygen • Pipeline • Cylinder • Storage • Failure • Delivery
- Simulation

KEY POINTS

- Continuous oxygen delivery is vital for safe anesthesia care.
- Oxygen supply failure is a potential crisis, and it is important to know it can occur and how to manage it.
- Understanding oxygen storage requirements, distribution, connections, and regulator and alarm functions is essential for managing supply failures.
- Simulation can successfully identify knowledge deficits and management difficulties during oxygen supply failures.
- Immediate management should focus on ensuring an oxygen supply, and maintaining oxygenation, ventilation, and anesthesia.

INTRODUCTION

Although uncommon, failures of the oxygen supply during anesthesia care are potentially life-threatening situations requiring an immediate and effective response.[1,2] Knowledge of the oxygen supply system, causes of failure, and the steps to remedy the failure are needed to address problems involving the oxygen supply.[3] Failures in the oxygen supply can occur at any point in the system, and the causes are numerous (**Table 1**). A 1997 American Society of Anesthesiologists (ASA) closed claims study of

[a] Department of Anesthesiology and Perioperative Medicine, Oregon Health and Science University, 3181 Southwest Sam Jackson Park Road, M/C SJH-2, Portland, OR 97239, USA; [b] Riverside Anesthesia Associates, Harrisburg, PA, USA; [c] University of Pittsburgh Medical Center (UPMC) Pinnacle, Harrisburg, PA, USA; [d] Department of Anesthesiology and Perioperative Medicine, Pennsylvania State University Hospital, Hershey, PA, USA; [e] Geisinger Health System, Danville, PA, USA; [f] Department of Anesthesiology and Perioperative Medicine, University of Texas MD Anderson Cancer Center–Houston, 1515 Holcombe Boulevard Unit 409, Houston, TX 77030, USA
[1] Present address: 60 Kirby Drive, Elizabethtown, PA 17022.
* Corresponding author.
E-mail address: botneyr@ohsu.edu
Twitter: @mdasandman (C.E.C.)

Anesthesiology Clin 38 (2020) 901–921
https://doi.org/10.1016/j.anclin.2020.08.005
1932-2275/20/© 2020 Elsevier Inc. All rights reserved.

anesthesiology.theclinics.com

Table 1
Reported causes of failures to supply oxygen

Category	Reported Examples
Lack of oxygen	Depletion of central or reserve supply during use[9,10] Emptied bulk liquid oxygen tank[11] Pipeline leaks or damage[2,9,12–14] Oxygen hose disconnections or misconnection from wall source[1,10]
Gases or substances other than oxygen	Tanks/cylinders filled with other gases[6,10,15] Tanks of other gases have oxygen fittings and are connected to bulk oxygen supply[16] Retrograde contamination from a nitrous oxide/oxygen blender[17] Water[18] or other contaminants in pipeline[19,20] Crossed pipeline in either the facility or the machine (may include failure of indexing systems or tampering)[3,4,6,7,9,10,21]
Low flow/obstructions to flow	Low system pressure Demand for flow exceeds system capacity[9] Compressed pipelines[9,22,23] Thermal damage to oxygen hose[9,24] Particulate matter from welding[9] Closed OR pipeline valve Regulator malfunction[9]
System shutdowns	Unannounced shutdowns[9,25]
Environmental causes	Frozen regulators, lightning damage[9] Tornados[26] Earthquakes[27]

Data from Refs.[1–4,6,7,9–27]

cases reported that 76% of claims involving gas delivery equipment resulted in death or brain damage, of which 11% resulted from problems with the oxygen supply.[4] A 2013 update reported no claims specific to the oxygen supply.[5] These changes may reflect improvements in warning systems and equipment, elimination of obsolete equipment, the development of guidelines and standards, and education. However, incidents involving the oxygen supply continue to occur.[6–8]

OXYGEN STORAGE AND DELIVERY

Oxygen is supplied to anesthesia machines from pipelines or machine-mounted cylinders. Oxygen supply systems include bulk oxygen supplies and backup cylinder banks, pipeline distribution, and associated monitoring. Oxygen and the entire supply system are subject to regulatory oversight and strict purity standards.

Oxygen Supply Oversight

Oxygen used in patient care is defined as a gas that is manufactured, packaged, and intended for administration to patients in anesthesia, or for therapy or diagnostic purposes.[28] The Federal Food, Drug, and Cosmetic Act provides for enforcement by federal and state agencies, including the Food and Drug Administration (FDA).[29] Standards for purity are published by the United States Pharmacopeia (USP).[30] The US Department of Transportation regulates medical gas cylinders and containers.[31]

Multiple additional authorities provide standards and guidelines, and the ASA has representation at many of them. The Compressed Gas Association (CGA) develops many of the safety standards used, and the American Society of Sanitary Engineers provides the oversight for gas plumbing. Codes for oxygen storage and delivery in hospitals and ambulatory facilities are found in the National Fire Protection Association (NFPA) 99 Health Care Facilities Code, hereafter referred to as NFPA 99.[32]

Oxygen Purity

Treatment or prevention of hypoxemia or hypoxia requires medical-grade oxygen that must adhere to Current Goods Manufacturing Processes (CGMP) as set forth by laws regulated by the FDA. The CGMP assures drug safety, identity, strength, quality, and purity. If oxygen is not handled according to these standards, then it is considered to be adulterated and not suitable for medical use. Medical gas manufacturing facilities must be certified to the "designated medical gas" requirements of the FDA.[29] Criteria for purity of medical-grade oxygen have been defined by USP standards. According to the CGMP, medical oxygen is labeled as "Oxygen USP" or "Oxygen 93 USP." USP standards require that "Oxygen USP" must meet or exceed 99% oxygen content, whereas "Oxygen 93 USP," produced by oxygen concentrators, has oxygen concentrations between 90.0% and 96.0%, with the remaining elements primarily argon and nitrogen.[30] Medical-grade oxygen cannot contain more than 0.001% of carbon monoxide and no more than 0.03% carbon dioxide; it should have no appreciable odor, and also be anhydrous, without any appreciable humidity.

Oxygen Storage

Oxygen may be stored as gas or liquid. Compressed gas cylinders are convenient to use, but their relatively small volume can necessitate frequent cylinder changes that introduce possible errors, decrease efficiency, and are not usually cost-effective.[6] Compressed oxygen cylinders can become dangerous projectiles if cylinder or valve damage occurs.[2] Liquid oxygen storage units are used when large amounts of oxygen are needed, eliminating the movement of heavy cylinders, decreasing costs, and simplifying gas delivery networks.[2,33]

In 2001, the FDA issued a Public Health Advisory to prevent delivery errors and contamination.[34] It recommended separate storage of medical-grade and industrial-grade gases, that personnel receive training specific to label recognition and for connecting containers to medical supply systems, emphasized that fittings on medical gas containers should not be changed under any condition, and that once a cryogenic container (used for storage of liquid oxygen) is attached to a system, a knowledgeable person should verify a proper connection.

Liquid Oxygen Storage Systems

Choosing what type of central oxygen supply to use depends on the number of beds, acuity of care, and peak demand.[9,11,35] The main types of central oxygen supplies are referred to as "liquid storage systems" and "liquid containers." Liquid storage systems are capable of much higher flows (3000 L/min) than those provided by liquid containers (500 L/min) and are therefore preferred for large facilities, whereas liquid containers are more suited to smaller sites.[33]

Bulk oxygen supplies frequently consist of cryogenic liquid storage (CLS) in large, anchored vessels known as vacuum insulated evaporators (VIE) (**Fig. 1**).[33,36] These tanks have an inner and outer lining separated by a vacuum to minimize heat transfer, and mechanisms to adjust for increases or decreases in internal pressure. The tanks are refilled from supply trucks on a regular schedule. NFPA 55 requires that the refill

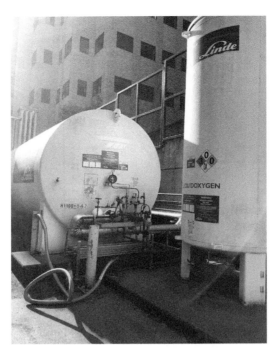

Fig. 1. Primary and secondary storage tanks for liquid oxygen. The primary tank (*left*) is significantly larger than the secondary tank (*right*).

location minimizes exposure to potential ignition sources by appropriate distancing from sidewalks, parked vehicles, and other objects.[37] Main oxygen supply branches should be isolated from sources of carbon monoxide, such as vehicle exhaust, back-up electrical generators, and other engines.

If the central oxygen supply is located outside the building it serves and 1 day's backup supply is not available, NFPA 99 requires an Emergency Oxygen Supply Connection fitting on the building's exterior with year-round access for connecting a temporary auxiliary supply source. An emergency backup supply located inside the building may be used in place of the connector.[32]

Smaller facilities may use liquid-filled containers, which are replaced by the supplier as the tanks are emptied.[16] Some facilities may use portable liquid oxygen tanks that do not exceed a capacity of 1.5 L and are managed similarly to portable gas cylinders. These portable liquid tanks are usually filled by clinical users.[31] The filling area should be treated like any area with an oxygen-enriched atmosphere, and precautions should be taken to eliminate fuel and ignition sources.

Cylinder Storage

Unlike many liquid *storage* systems, cylinders used to *supply* oxygen are often stored inside. If stored outside, they must be protected from extremes in temperature variation.[31,38] Two common cylinder sizes are the E cylinder, which is used on anesthesia machines or for patient transport and holds about 660 L of oxygen at a pressure of about 2000 psi, and the larger H cylinder, which contains 6900 L of oxygen at 2200 psi.[31,39,40]

According to NFPA 99, cylinders that are in use must be placed in a stand or designated cylinder holder and not chained to portable objects, such as beds or stretchers, nor stored in operating rooms (ORs).[32] Cylinders that are in use in the OR are not considered to be in storage. Storage locations must prevent unauthorized entry and must be constructed from either noncombustible or limited-combustible materials. Oxygen and other oxidizing gases must be stored separately from flammable agents in a manner consistent with NFPA code, and smoking is prohibited in or around storage areas. Cylinders must be secured, with caps, in the upright position, for example, in racks designed to hold smaller cylinders, or secured with a chain (larger cylinders). Oxygen should be segregated from cylinders with different gases or nonmedical cylinders, and full cylinders must be separated from those that are empty.[2,38–40]

Ambulatory Centers and Office-Based Anesthesia

Free-standing ambulatory surgical centers and offices that perform anesthesia often use compressed gas cylinders of varying sizes as their oxygen supply source. Some larger centers with higher oxygen requirements may use liquid oxygen containers as their primary supply.[32,41,42]

Oxygen Concentrators

Oxygen concentrators are an alternative to the bulk storage of oxygen and can be used in a variety of settings, including small facilities. Air is passed through a molecular sieve containing zeolite granules. Using a process known as Pressure Swing Adsorption, nitrogen, carbon dioxide, carbon monoxide, water vapor, and hydrocarbons are adsorbed and removed, while oxygen and argon pass through, producing oxygen and argon. They produce Oxygen 93 USP and deliver oxygen with flows up to 10 L/min at an Fio_2 of about 95%.[35] They provide a cost-effective alternative that can be used as the sole oxygen supply, or added to an existing system as either a secondary or backup supply.

Large-scale concentrators can supply pipeline systems for routine use and as a backup. A pressurized reservoir large enough to meet peak flow requirements is required, which also provides protection against temporary electrical failure. It can be supplied by several concentrators connected in parallel. Any drop in reservoir pressure brings one or more concentrators into use until pressure is restored. A backup system is still required in case of malfunction or drop in oxygen concentration.

Although concentrators have certain advantages in cost savings, reliability, simplicity, and filtration of contaminants, some disadvantages and hazards are associated with their use. Regular cleaning of air intake filters is required; concentrators cannot produce 100% oxygen, and Fio_2 is further reduced in very high-humidity environments. If the air intake is contaminated by fumes, water, or other pollutants, the sieve medium could be damaged and prematurely exhausted. Oxygen concentrations can vary with gas flow, and in anesthesia circle breathing systems with low oxygen flows (<0.5 L/min) or closed circuits, argon concentrations greater than 5% may occur and decrease Fio_2, making oxygen concentration monitoring essential.[31]

Delivery Systems for Oxygen: Getting Oxygen from the Storage Unit to the Patient

Delivery of oxygen to anesthetized patients takes place in essentially 2 stages: (1) from the storage unit throughout the facility, and (2) from the pipeline or cylinder supply through the anesthesia machine to the patient.

As facility size and oxygen demand increase, supply systems become more complex, but commonalities exist in nearly all systems. A backup supply is often placed in a different area from the primary and secondary supplies and should enter the facility via a different route.[1,11] Liquid oxygen from the VIE passes through a vaporizer to generate oxygen gas, and a high-pressure regulator reduces the pressure. A subsequent regulator reduces gas pressure to 50 psi, after which oxygen enters the facility through the main pipeline. The pipeline splits into risers that extend vertically into the building to bring oxygen to each floor and supply the branch lines that run throughout each floor. Pipeline dimensions are chosen to minimize pressure drops from the source to the point of use. However, with increased flow through the pipeline and resultant frictional loss of pressure along the pipeline, it is possible for pressure to reduce sufficiently to affect equipment operation.[39]

Pipelines are critical components of the oxygen supply. Materials suitable for oxygen piping are specified in ASTM B819 and NFPA 99 and must be resistant to rust, leakage, or contamination; often copper is used as the pipeline material.[43] Any interconnection between pipelines for different gases is prohibited.[32] Construction and maintenance services for medical gas plumbing systems should be performed by qualified, competent technicians specialized in medical gas plumbing and certified to the most current standards. Ventilator and anesthesia machine failures have been reported secondary to particulate contamination from improper gas plumbing.[44] The NFPA requires both the installer and the user to corroborate the pipeline's completeness before patient use.

Central supply systems have a variety of mandated safety devices. A main valve at the primary source to the supply line is required. Pressure relief valves and one-way check valves are used throughout the piping system. Shutoff valves allow for isolation of different parts of the pipeline if a problem such as a leak or pipeline damage occurs or if service is required. Shutoff valves include source shutoff valves, a main line shutoff valve, riser, branch line, and zone shutoff valves. Any line that serves a patient care area must have a shutoff valve and a pressure gauge. Separate shutoff valves are required for anesthetizing locations where moderate sedation, deep sedation, or general anesthesia is provided. Shutoff valves for anesthetizing locations are designed with a 90° long-handled valve, which prevents replacement of the cover if the valve is in the closed position, should be within a box that has an easily removable window large enough to permit manual operation, and located near anesthetizing rooms, vital life-support, and critical care areas (**Fig. 2**). Ideally, those working in the area should know where shutoff valves are located before the need for use; many facilities have successfully integrated the location of these valves in their preprocedure checklist. In emergency situations, such as a fire or catastrophic equipment failure, the valves should be turned to the OFF position upon leaving the room or affected area.

Medical gas distribution systems must have warning systems to indicate failure. A master alarm system and gauges monitor the source supply of all gases, the backup supplies, and the pressure of each main line. Primary and secondary tanks should have low-pressure alarms to indicate when the main vessel supply is low, and to indicate when secondary and backup supplies are accessed. Alarms must notify both hospital maintenance/engineering and an area that is staffed 24 hours a day, such as a telephone switchboard. Alarms in the main supply line should alert when pressure varies by ±20% from normal pressure; alarms also activate when pressure variations (±20%) occur downstream from the main line (**Fig. 3**) or in cases of concentrator malfunction. Pressure alarms should be periodically tested.

Some facilities still provide oxygen solely from cylinder banks or free-standing cylinders (FSC) without a backup supply.[45] The cylinder banks are connected to manifolds or high-pressure header systems, which convert them into a single continuous supply. The primary cylinder bank is the one currently running, and the secondary

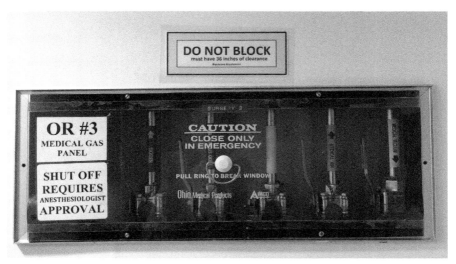

Fig. 2. Shut-off valves for an OR. The panel is located immediately outside the OR. Note that each valve is labeled and color-coded.

system is the standby supply. Check valves are used between each cylinder and the header to prevent loss of gas if there is a leak from a cylinder.

SAFETY MECHANISMS

Numerous safety mechanisms help ensure reliable and safe oxygen delivery. These safety mechanisms include the use of color-coding, specific connectors for different gases, engineered safety devices that help prevent delivery of hypoxic gas mixtures, oxygen analyzers, and various alarms. The use of all these mechanisms, although not guaranteeing oxygen supply and delivery, markedly reduce the risk that a hypoxic gas mixture would be delivered because of a failure of the oxygen supply. Notwithstanding the value of the mechanisms described above, knowledge of the anesthesia machine

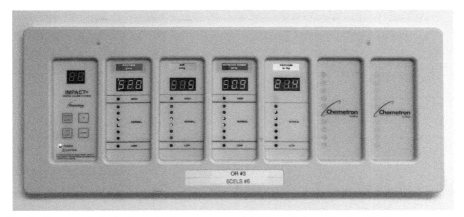

Fig. 3. Gas panel displaying pipeline pressures (*right*) and alarm testing (*left*).

and its preuse checkout is arguably the most important step for improving oxygen supply safety.

Components of an Anesthesia Machine and Preuse Checkout

Over time, the anesthesia machine has grown progressively more complex, and ISO 80601-2-13:2011 is the design standard used to ensure anesthesia machine safety.[46] However, oxygen supply systems have remained largely unchanged.

Oxygen serves several functions within an anesthesia machine.[47] Besides delivering an inhaled anesthetic to the patient, it supplies other components, such as the auxiliary flowmeter and oxygen flush valve, serves as a ventilator drive gas, powers the fail-safe mechanism, and, when absent, triggers the low oxygen pressure alarm.

Found on most anesthesia machines, the auxiliary flowmeter provides a route separate from the common gas outlet and the anesthesia circuit for oxygen delivery. Because the auxiliary flowmeter uses the same source of oxygen as the machine, if an issue of supply failure or adulteration arises, this flowmeter will have the same issue.

Flush valves deliver high, unmetered flows of oxygen directly to the common gas outlet from the oxygen source without passing through any other anesthesia machine components. The oxygen supplied to the flush valve is at pipeline or regulated cylinder pressures, at flow rates between 35 and 75 L/min[31] The flush valve functions independently of machine power.

Some machines use electrically powered piston or turbine ventilators to compress and drive inspired gases into the lungs without consuming oxygen, but many ventilators require a method referred to as pneumatic drive to deliver gas into the lungs. This method consumes a significant quantity of oxygen. If oxygen is being supplied from an E cylinder, it will only last between 30 and 90 minutes when used in such a system.[48,49]

The fail-safe device is an engineered safety mechanism that helps to prevent delivery of a hypoxic gas mixture. Whereas oxygen and air pass directly to their flowmeters, nitrous oxide must pass through a fail-safe device before reaching its flowmeter. This device is designed to interrupt the flow of nitrous oxide when oxygen supply pressure drops below a threshold value. The threshold pressure needed to activate the fail-safe mechanism is usually 20 psi.[31]

The low oxygen pressure alarm within the anesthesia machine is usually triggered when pressure within the machine decreases to less than 30 psi. Some older machines use a Ritchie Whistle, which creates a distinct audible alarm.[50] Newer machines use electronic alarms, which rely on electrical power to function.

Oxygen analyzers measure the Fio_2 in the breathing circuit. Mazze[10] called for their routine use, stating, "[w]hile they will not prevent delivery of a hypoxic gas mixture, they help to eliminate reliance on human performance to prevent or detect problems with oxygen delivery." ASA monitoring standards require oxygen analyzers for the detection of hypoxic gas mixtures.[51] Contemporary oxygen analyzers have an alarm that cannot be permanently silenced.

Because oxygen flow is dependent on electrical power, the machine should have a nondetachable power cord plugged into a red-colored outlet (for emergency generator backup), along with a backup battery capable of sustaining power for at least 30 minutes. Significant variability exists among anesthesia machines. For example, some machines display oxygen pipeline and cylinder pressures on mechanical gauges that are always visible, whereas newer machines display these pressures electronically, but only during machine checkout (**Fig. 4**). Having information such as this always visible and easily accessible can be beneficial during an oxygen supply failure.[31]

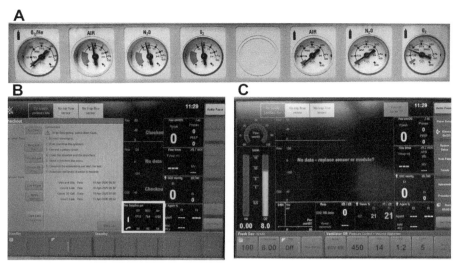

Fig. 4. Cylinder pressures displayed on different anesthesia machines. (*A*) Mechanical pressure gauges on anesthesia machines are always visible. (*B*) On an electronic display, cylinder pressures are visible in the yellow highlighted section of the display, but only during machine checkout. (*C*) Cylinder pressures are no longer displayed once checkout is complete.

An anesthesia machine's preuse checkout is performed to confirm the machine's ability to perform its intended functions, including reliably delivering oxygen. Understanding machine design helps understand which steps in the checkout process are important for oxygen delivery. In contemporary machines, many of these steps are now automated and no longer performed manually. The manner in which steps are done varies with the manufacturer and model of the machine. Steps important for oxygen delivery are identified in **Box 1**.

Color-Coding

Although medical gas cylinders are color-coded for easy identification, reading the label is considered the definitive method for identifying a cylinder's contents. See **Box 2** and **Fig. 5** for information that is displayed on the cylinder label.[31] Because color-

---

Box 1
Steps in the machine checkout that are important for verifying oxygen delivery

Verify presence of self-inflating bag (SIB)

Confirm pipeline pressure of 50 psi, and cylinder pressure at least 1000 psi

Perform leak test of low-pressure part of the machine

Check calibration of oxygen analyzer

Test flowmeter function, including oxygen/nitrous oxide proportioning system

Confirm function of fail-safe mechanism and oxygen supply pressure alarm

Check scavenging system positive and negative pressure relief valve function

Perform positive pressure leak test of breathing circuit assembly

Confirm ventilator and unidirectional valves function correctly

---

Box 2
Information that may be displayed on a gas cylinder label

Name of gas

Diamond shape denoting hazard class for the contained gas:
• Oxidizer
• Nonflammable gas
• Flammable gas

Signal word indicating level of hazard to health or property, dangers associated with handling or use, and measures to avoid injury or damage:
• Danger (immediate)
• Warning (less than immediate)
• Caution (not immediate)

Cylinder maker/distributor name and address

Volume (in liters) at 70°F

Expiration date for contents

---

coding is not a universal standard, mixups because of differences in color-coding have led to fatal errors.[6] Nonetheless, color-coding can contribute to safety and is used ubiquitously throughout the anesthesia machine and oxygen supply system. In addition to oxygen cylinders, pipelines, gauges, valves, hoses, connectors, flowmeters, and knobs use color-coding. In the United States, green is designated as the color for medical oxygen cylinders and requires that at least the shoulder of the compressed gas cylinder be colored to represent the compressed gas it contains, with it visible when looking from above.[52] Internationally, white is used for medical oxygen cylinders.[39]

Connectors

The CGA has written standards to prevent cross-connections and misconnection of medical gases and so reduce the possibility of inadvertent substitution of medical gases.[53] In the United States, supply system connections use the American Standard Safety System for gas cylinders with volumes exceeding 25 cubic feet (707 L). Smaller containers, such as E cylinders, use the pin index safety system (PISS), and wall fittings and those on the back of the machine use the diameter index safety system (DISS). There are also quick release systems, such as Schrader, Chemetron, Ohio Diamond, and Puritan valves, which are unique to each manufacturer.

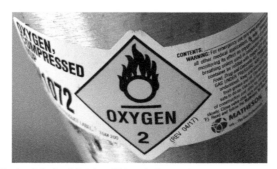

Fig. 5. Oxygen cylinder label with identifying information.

DISS connectors are used where the hoses attach to the anesthesia machine and for some wall connections (**Fig. 6**). A threaded nut is permanently affixed to the hose, and a threaded receiver is located on the wall or machine connection. To prevent connection errors, the bore diameters and bolt thread are unique to each medical gas. Quick connect/disconnect systems are used for some wall and ceiling mount connections of gas hoses to the pipeline supply (**Fig. 7**).

Compressed gas cylinders with volumes less than 25 cubic feet, such as an E cylinder, use a PISS connection. Pins are placed in indexed locations, which differ for each type of gas cylinder. Yokes have a gas orifice and 2 pins that occupy 2 of 6 possible positions. Cylinders have holes on the valve body. Cylinders will only properly seat on a yoke when a pin-hole connection is achieved. For example, oxygen yokes use pins in the number 2 and number 5 positions (commonly referred to as the 2–5 pin index), and only a cylinder with holes bored in the 2 and 5 locations fit the oxygen yoke (**Fig. 8**). Pin indexing systems are also found on regulators and filling systems.

Regulators

*Regulators are an essential component that is used in numerous locations within the oxygen supply system, including liquid storage containers, gas cylinders, pipeline networks, and anesthesia machines. Regulators reduce pressures that could damage equipment or pipelines, provide a constant pressure output to facilitate proper equipment function, and allow multiple sources of gas to be connected, such as the pipeline and cylinder supplies in the machine. Oxygen regulators are susceptible to damage, freezing, or other failures, which may lead to excess pressures or interruptions to the oxygen supply.[54]

Alarms

Alarms attract attention to a specific abnormality, typically with a sound and visual indicator. Because alarm systems can become disconnected or fail to sound, they should be checked periodically. The professional must identify the source of the

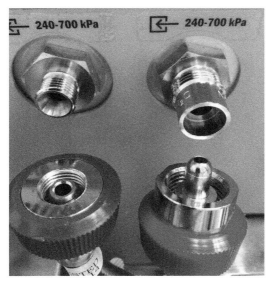

Fig. 6. DISS connections for oxygen and nitrous oxide.

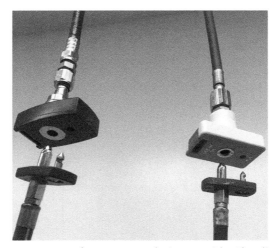

Fig. 7. Quick-release connectors for oxygen and nitrous oxide. The diameter of the hose connectors differs, as does the spacing between them, preventing misconnections.

"interrupt," determine the nature of the alarming condition, evaluate the context, and determine a response.[55] If the alarm is related to a problem with the oxygen supply, it requires a deliberate and immediate response.[9,25]

SIMULATION AND CRISIS MANAGEMENT

Because gas delivery equipment problems are rare, prospective studies are difficult. Simulation offers an opportunity to study responses to oxygen supply failures and appears to be an important aid for learning management of these critical incidents. Two different scenarios have been studied: the loss of pipeline oxygen supply and the

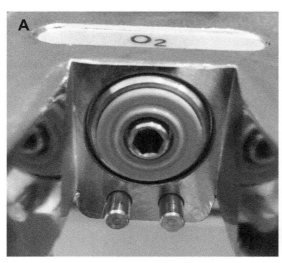
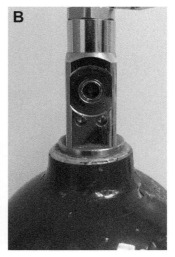

Fig. 8. PISS for oxygen. (*A*) Pin indexing for the oxygen yoke. (*B*) Corresponding holes for an oxygen cylinder.

crossed pipeline connection, which results in a lack of oxygen delivery despite the appearance that there is oxygen supply pressure and flow. Simulations of the loss of oxygen supply have demonstrated major gaps in performance and knowledge (**Box 3**).[14,56–60] There are similar lessons to be learned from a simulation of crossed pipeline connections, including deficits in understanding machine design and function, and that equipment design can contribute to difficulties in management. The investigators note that the "participants' lack of knowledge of the anesthesia machine and gas supply, coupled with complexity and shortfalls in equipment design, particularly with regard to alarms and other safety functions, led to suboptimal management of a potentially lethal crisis."[61]

Box 3
Observations and lessons learned from simulation of loss of oxygen supply

Poor understanding of oxygen supply failure

Lack of plans for safe and effective management

Failures to identify empty oxygen cylinder during machine checkout

Poor understanding of anesthesia machine and oxygen supply

Difficulties with reserve cylinders:
• Inability to open reserve cylinder
• Difficulty replacing reserve cylinder

Poor conservation of oxygen cylinder supply:
• Use low flows
• Close adjustable pressure limiting (APL) valve
• Switch to manual ventilation (if oxygen used as ventilator drive gas)

Failures to maintain anesthetic, with risk of patient awareness

Failures to verify oxygen purity before resuming use of pipeline supply

Recommend using written protocols and standardized responses

FAILURE MODALITIES AND MANAGEMENT

Any attempt at understanding failures to supply oxygen and subsequent management requires detailed knowledge of how oxygen is supplied. Problems with oxygen delivery can involve storage, distribution, or problems with the pipeline and/or cylinder supply to the anesthesia machine, or the internal workings of the machine. However, machine problems affecting oxygen delivery, such as internal leaks, flowmeter malfunctions, problems with the oxygen/nitrous oxide proportioning or fail-safe mechanisms, or breathing circuit or ventilator issues, when the oxygen supply is otherwise intact, are outside the scope of this section and are not addressed here.

Supply failures can be limited in their extent, readily addressed, and quickly resolved, or they can affect the entire facility for a substantial period of time and have an impact on operations.[1,11] Reported failures of the oxygen supply have been listed in **Table 1**; some important considerations are discussed later in greater detail.

Problems with the Bulk Oxygen Supply

Problems with the bulk oxygen supply range from depletion of oxygen or low pressure for other reasons to contamination or filling of the supply container with something other than oxygen. Depletion can occur because of high levels of use, and although many systems have a secondary supply, that can also be depleted, with the backup supply eventually running out, too. Because of redundancies in the stored supply, this should be a rare occurrence. There can also be a loss of oxygen because of failure of the equipment associated with oxygen storage, including valves, regulators, and piping coming off the tank, resulting in a loss of oxygen and drop in system pressure. The low-pressure alarm usually provides notice of this problem, although some systems also monitor container volume.

Contamination of the bulk supply by air, nitrogen, or other gases has been reported. Contamination can occur because tanks or cylinders have been filled with gases other than oxygen, or because tanks of other gases have been connected to the bulk oxygen supply.[6,10,15,16] Such events are typically detected by a drop in Fio_2 on the oxygen analyzer.

If the oxygen supply has excessively high pressures, a high-pressure alarm is triggered. Equipment can be damaged, including storage containers and the pipeline, and barotrauma may result. If damage occurs, it may affect the oxygen supply pressure and flow. Increases in pipeline pressure can occur if there is a regulator failure in the central oxygen supply, if the regulator is set higher in order to compensate for low system pressures, or as a result from combustion of foreign material in the pipeline.[9,31,54]

Problems with the Pipeline

Pipeline distribution networks tend to be rather complex, and the more complex the system, the greater the opportunity for failure. In addition to supply failures, low pressures can result from pipeline leaks or high demand. Alarms involving gas panels in the OR should generate a response by anesthesia staff. Leaks occur during pipeline work, including construction, remodeling, or maintenance, or from other construction work within the facility that damages pipelines. If the pressure failure occurs because of damage or failure of gas piping, the area in question should be isolated and bypassed for repairs. Obstructions to flow can also interfere with pipeline delivery of oxygen. In some cases, valves have been closed and flow shut off to sections of the pipeline, either accidentally or without proper notice.

Contamination can occur when a different substance is present in the oxygen pipeline that is not due to crossed connections. Particulate matter, water, and introduction of air or other substances in the pipeline have been reported.[17–20] A contaminant may not cause an alarm condition at all, unless it is present in sufficient quantity to reduce Fio_2, in which case the oxygen analyzer and gas monitor should alarm.

A special class of pipeline contamination is the crossed connection, usually involving nitrous oxide and oxygen pipelines, and commonly seen in new facilities, or after construction (ie, new ORs are built or new pipelines are added to existing systems), after maintenance work on the pipeline system or, in rare cases, as a result of deliberate tampering. Crossed connections will manifest with an oxygen analyzer that reads very low. The gas monitor should also show a low inspiratory oxygen level but, in addition, an unexpectedly high level of nitrous oxide, if that is the other gas involved in the crossed connection. However, gas flows will appear intact. Finally, the pulse oximeter will start to demonstrate a low oxygen saturation, but again, this will typically be a late finding.

Problems with Connections Involving the Anesthesia Machine

DISS and other connections can fail in several ways. Hoses can be intentionally unplugged, or connectors may fail, thus preventing gas flow.[10] Obstructions can occur by hoses becoming trapped under a wheel of a machine or getting pinched off in some other way.[22,23] Hoses can rupture and leak because of age, or because of other effects, such as thermal damage.[24] Such problems manifest as low supply pressure, although they can occur intermittently.[23] A loss of supply pressure will be reflected by a lack of oxygen flow, and with the fail-safe mechanism operative, a lack of nitrous oxide flow, as well. The pipeline pressure gauge will read zero, the ventilator bellows may not refill completely (assuming mechanical ventilation), and the oxygen analyzer will be trending down.

Another significant issue is when the hose is plugged into another gas' connector, another form of crossed connections. Usually this occurs when the wrong connector has been attached to the oxygen hose or installed at the pipeline outlet. If this happens, the oxygen analyzer will display a low Fio_2; however, it may not manifest until late in the case, when the "oxygen" flow is turned up and other gases are turned off, if another gas is misconnected to the oxygen line. A similar crossed connection can occur with piping inside the anesthesia machine, usually following machine maintenance.

Alarms may originate from the oxygen analyzer, a gas monitor, the oxygen supply pressure monitor, or the pulse oximeter, and the immediate response will be from anesthesia staff. Evaluation of these devices should indicate the nature of the problem, whether it is a loss of supply pressure, crossed connections, or some other perturbation of the oxygen supply.

Loss of Cylinder Supply

The cylinder is used as a backup oxygen supply in most cases, although it may be the machine's primary oxygen source if a pipeline supply is not available. The cylinder requires a wrench or key to open and close the cylinder valve. A pressure gauge displays cylinder pressure, and a regulator reduces pressure to 45 psi, slightly less than pipeline pressure, so that the pipeline is the preferred source under normal operating conditions. After checkout, the cylinder can remain open or be closed. The argument for leaving it open is that in case of pipeline failure, it can immediately provide oxygen without any interruption to its delivery. However, this is a dangerous practice. If there is a pipeline failure, the low-pressure alarm will not sound and the provider will be unaware it has occurred until the cylinder empties, at which point there is no oxygen available. The cylinder could empty because of a poor hose connection, or because pipeline pressures can go lower than the regulated cylinder pressure, intermittently making it the primary source of oxygen, thus gradually emptying the cylinder.[10,22] Given the reported difficulties in replacing a cylinder, especially in stressful situations, such as loss of the oxygen supply, closing the cylinder valve after machine checkout is recommended.

Management of Oxygen Supply Failures

Optimal management consists of 4 basic principles: (1) ensure the oxygen supply, (2) maintain oxygenation, (3) maintain ventilation, and (4) maintain the anesthetic.

The first, and possibly most important step in managing oxygen supply failure, is preventing it from occurring. Preventative steps include those that can reduce the likelihood of a supply interruption in the first place or ensuring that if there is a failure involving some portion of the system, that uninterrupted supply of oxygen nonetheless continues. Many of these preventative measures address what are known as latent errors, defined as potential failure modes that are present throughout the system, hidden from view and remaining dormant until conditions exist that, in combination with other system flaws, thwart system defenses, resulting in an adverse event.[62] Latent errors are readily identifiable in reports of oxygen supply failures.

One preventative measure involves ongoing monitoring of the supply system; this could include a daily audit of oxygen consumption, which may use continuous measurement of CLS contents to assess whether the central source is filled with the correct gas and has adequate volume. Alarms for low volume and excessive rate of volume loss can help with this. The availability of adequate secondary and backup supplies, and automatic switching to these supplies, should be confirmed.

Installation of new pipelines, routine maintenance, renovations, or modification to any part of the oxygen supply and delivery system should be considered special risks for disruption of oxygen supply. At a minimum, pipelines should be flushed, pressures checked, and gas composition analyzed and certified at these times.

Finally, system components should be protected from damage. Consider either a physical or spatial barrier between primary and secondary tanks, so that damage to one does not impair use of the other, and use independent pipelines from each tank into the facility.[1,11,63] Feedlines connecting source containers to the facility should incorporate design features, such as shielding and prominent labeling, to prevent accidental interruptions, for example, during street repairs.

Ensuring proper equipment function is key to being able to effectively manage and mitigate a supply failure. Complete and thorough daily machine checks, including filling status of the backup cylinder and presence of an SIB, are essential. These checks should include confirmation that the pipeline is connected and at proper pressure, the cylinder has been closed, no leaks are present, and flowmeters and monitors function properly. Monitors and alarms should be used; they should not be broken, silenced, or ignored. Using nonpneumatically driven ventilators, or using air as the drive gas, will limit consumption of oxygen in event of a supply loss.

Contingency planning is important and can take place at either the anesthesia department or the OR level, or involve the entire facility. Simulations can help prepare anesthesia providers to manage these crisis situations, while disaster planning for supply system failures, including mock drills, can be part of the facility's preparedness. The backup system should have sufficient capacity to meet needs until a truck arrives to replenish the central supply, while an external emergency connection from the supply truck to the central system can provide oxygen to the facility upon its arrival. The facility should also have an adequate supply of cylinders to meet its needs in the event of a system failure.

Presentation of an Event

There are several ways by which a provider can recognize that a problem has developed with the oxygen supply. The exact manner in which a failure presents will depend on the type of event, whether low pressure and loss of the oxygen supply or the presence of a gas other than oxygen in the supply.

If a loss of oxygen occurs, the preuse checkout may fail. It can be recognized during anesthesia when the low supply pressure, oxygen analyzer, gas monitor, or pulse oximeter alarms sound, and pressure gauges display a loss of oxygen pressure. Apnea alarms may sound because of low ventilator pressures and tidal volumes, and absent end-tidal CO_2. There are several indications that flow has been lost, including lack of flow in the flowmeters or flush valve, and an oxygen-driven ventilator ceases function. There may be an audible sound if a hose is disconnected from the pipeline or is leaking.

If there is a gas other than oxygen within the oxygen supply, early recognition is from low oxygen levels on the oxygen analyzer or gas monitor. High levels of the substituted gas, for example, nitrous oxide, may also be displayed on the gas monitor. Low oxygen or high nitrous oxide alarms may sound. Subsequently, the pulse oximeter displays low oxygen saturation and also alarms. There may be clinical signs, as well, such as cyanosis or rhythm disturbances.

Immediate Management

When presented with a failure of the oxygen supply, the cause is not usually immediately obvious, beyond a problem with oxygenation. It may be quickly recognized and fixed, for example, the hose had been disconnected from the pipeline and the cylinder has emptied, in which case the solution is to reconnect the hose back to the pipeline. Often the problem is not quickly identified and quickly resolved, and management is much more complex, for example, disruption of the oxygen pipeline elsewhere in the facility, with loss of oxygen to many locations for an indeterminate period of time. Whatever the exact cause, the immediate objective is to maintain oxygenation, ventilation, and anesthesia. In all but the simplest of situations, these are accomplished with an oxygen source, a method for positive pressure ventilation, and either continuation of the inhaled agent or switching to an intravenous (IV) anesthetic (**Table 2**).

Oxygen can be provided by the cylinder on the machine or a FSC with a regulator. The exact choice of which to use may rely on the individual situation. For example, if an FSC is not immediately available, the obvious first choice is to open the backup

Table 2
Immediate actions to take for any oxygen supply failure

Oxygen Source	Immediate Actions		
	Machine Cylinder	**Free-Standing Cylinder**	**Room Air**
To oxygenate	Open cylinder	Open cylinder	N/A
To ventilate	Use breathing circuit	Use self-inflating bag	Use self-inflating bag
CALL FOR HELP			
Pipeline	Check pressure gauge, disconnect from wall		
Anesthetic	Inhaled	IV	IV
Confirm oxygenation	Check: • Cylinder pressure gauge • Oxygen analyzer Fio_2 • Gas monitor Fio_2 • Flowmeters have gas flow	Connect elbow adaptor with its gas monitor connection Check gas monitor Fio_2	N/A (can connect elbow adaptor with gas monitor connection to confirm $EtCO_2$)
Conserve oxygen	• Reduce oxygen flow to minimum necessary • Close APL valve • Use manual ventilation (unless oxygen not used as ventilator drive gas)	Reduce cylinder flow to minimum needed	N/A
INFORM SURGEON			
STABILIZE PATIENT			

Color legend: Red: urgent priorities; green: oxygen-related; yellow: air-related; brown: additional priorities.

machine cylinder and oxygenate using the machine circuit. Alternatively, a temporary measure would be to use an SIB and room air. If an FSC is available, use it with a Jackson-Reese or SIB to maintain oxygenation and ventilation. Keep in mind that if the machine cylinder is not used, an IV anesthetic will have to be started. This is an excellent time to call for help.

Several additional actions should also be promptly done. If a loss of supply is suspected, check the pipeline gauge to confirm pressure has dropped. The hose should be disconnected from the pipeline, especially if a gas other than oxygen is suspected. Oxygenation should be confirmed by checking the cylinder pressure gauge to confirm it has oxygen, the oxygen analyzer, and gas monitor to confirm Fio_2, and flowmeters to confirm flow. If using an FSC, the elbow adaptor and gas monitor connection can be used to confirm Fio_2. Steps to conserve oxygen should also be taken at this time, by reducing oxygen flow to the minimum necessary, closing the APL valve (if using the machine cylinder), and switching to manual ventilation (unless oxygen is not used to drive the ventilator). The surgeon must be informed.

Subsequent Management Steps

Once the patient has been stabilized, additional steps should be taken. Notify the OR and facility staff about the problem and ascertain the extent and expected duration of the failure. Knowledge of the extent and expected duration may influence planning for obtaining additional oxygen supplies and whether surgeries need to be discontinued or postponed. Additional oxygen cylinders should be obtained, for the machine or free-standing. If oxygen supply runs out, it may be necessary to use room air with an SIB or spontaneous ventilation; oxygen may need to be prioritized to patients needing an Fio_2 greater than room air. Additional supplies for IV anesthesia may be needed. It may be necessary to attend to complications or unstable patients. Before resuming pipeline use, testing should confirm the composition (oxygen, not another gas) and quality (without contaminants) of the gas. In extreme situations, it may be necessary to arrange transfer of patients to other facilities. Once the event is over, a critical incident report should be completed. Debriefing of patients may be necessary.

DISCLOSURE

R. Botney has nothing to disclose. J.F. Answine has nothing to disclose. C.E. Cowles, Technical Committee Member for National Fire Protection Association (NFPA) Healthcare Section. Travel expense reimbursement only.

REFERENCES

1. Herff H, Paal P, von Goedecke A, et al. Fatal errors in nitrous oxide delivery. Anaesthesia 2007;62:1202–6.
2. Mostert L, Coetzee AR. Central oxygen supply failure. South Afr J Anaesth Analg 2014;20:214–7.
3. Petty W. AANA journal course: update for nurse anesthetists-medical gases, hospital pipelines, and medical gas cylinders: how safe are they? AANA J 1995;63:307–24.
4. Caplan R, Vistica M, Posner K, et al. Adverse anesthetic outcomes arising from gas delivery equipment: a closed claims analysis. Anest 1997;87:741–8.
5. Mehta SP, Eisenkraft JB, Posner KL, et al. Patient injuries from anesthesia gas delivery equipment: a closed claims update. Anest 2013;119:788–95.

6. Pauling M, Ball CM. Delivery of anoxic gas mixtures in anaesthesia: case report and review of the struggle towards safer standards of care. Anaesth Intensive Care 2017;45:21–8.

7. Dangoisse MJ, Lalot M, Lechat JP. Connection error in the delivery of medical gases to a surgical unit. Acta Anaesthesiol Belg 2010;61:33–7.

8. Gilfor JM, Ehrenworth J. Nitrogen contamination of operating room oxygen pipeline. APSF Newsletter 2019;34:25–6. Available at: https://www.apsf.org/newsletter/june-2019/. Accessed February 26, 2020.

9. Feeley TW, Hedley-Whyte J. Bulk oxygen and nitrous oxide delivery systems: design and dangers. Anest 1976;44:301–5.

10. Mazze RI. Therapeutic misadventures with oxygen delivery systems: the need for continuous in-line oxygen monitors. Anesth Analg 1972;51:787–92.

11. Schumacher SD, Brockwell RC, Andrews JJ, et al. Bulk liquid oxygen supply failure. Anest 2004;100:186–9.

12. Black AE. Extraordinary oxygen pipeline failure: a coping strategy. Anaesthesia 1990;45:599–600.

13. Lacoumenta S, Hall GM. A burst oxygen pipeline. Anaesthesia 1983;38:596–7.

14. Weller J, Merry A, Warman G, et al. Anaesthetists' management of oxygen pipeline failure: room for improvement. Anaesthesia 2007;62:122–6.

15. Sprague DH, Archer GW Jr. Intraoperative hypoxia from an erroneously filled liquid oxygen reservoir. Anest 1975;42:360–2.

16. Bernstein DB, Rosenberg AD. Intraoperative hypoxia from nitrogen tanks with oxygen fittings. Anesth Analg 1997;84:225–7.

17. Lye A, Patrick R. Oxygen contamination of the nitrous oxide pipeline supply. Anaesth Intensive Care 1998;26:207–9.

18. Hay H. Contamination of piped medical gas supply with water. Eur J Anaesth 2000;17:512–4.

19. Eichhorn JH, Bancroft ML, Laasberg LH, et al. Contamination of medical gas and water pipelines in a new hospital building. Anest 1977;46:286–9.

20. Gilmour IJ, McComb RC, Palahniuk RJ. Contamination of a hospital oxygen supply. Anesth Analg 1990;71:302–4.

21. Scamman FL. An analysis of factors leading to crossed gas lines causing profound hypercarbia during general anesthesia. J Clin Anesth 1993;5:439–41.

22. Anderson WR, Brock-Utne JG. Oxygen pipeline supply failure: a coping strategy. J Clin Monit 1991;7:39–41.

23. Williams D. Occlusion of oxygen pipeline supply. Anaesth Intensive Care 1999;27:221–2.

24. Ewart IA. An unusual cause of gas pipeline failure. Anaesthesia 1990;45:498.

25. Gjerde GE. Retrograde pressurization of a medical oxygen pipeline system: safety backup or hazard? Crit Care Med 1980;8:219–21.

26. Johnson DL. Central oxygen supply versus mother nature. Respir Care 1975;20:1043–4.

27. Los Angeles Times. Hospitals hold up, but services shut down. Jan 20, 1994; p. B1, B4.

28. CGA G-4. Oxygen. Arlington (VA): Compressed Gas Association, Inc; 2015.

29. Code of Federal Regulations, Title 21 CFR (Food and Drugs). Washington, DC: U.S. Government Printing Office.

30. United States Pharmacopeia. Pharmacopeial Forum 2005; 31(4):1107. Rockville, MD.

31. Dorsch JA, Dorsch SE. Medical gas cylinders and containers. In: Understanding anesthesia equipment. 5th edition. Philadelphia: Lippincott Williams & Wilkins; 2008. p. 1–22.
32. National Fire Protection Association. Health care facilities code (NFPA 99). Quincy (MA): 2018.
33. Bland H, Borton C, Jafri S. The supply of anaesthetic and other medical gasses. In: Davey AJ, Diba A, editors. Ward's Anaesthetic equipment. 6th edition. Edinburgh (Scotland): Saunders Elsevier; 2012. p. 1–26.
34. Guidance for hospitals, nursing homes, and other health care facilities. FDA Public Health Advisory. 2001. Available at: https://www.fda.gov/files/drugs/published/Guidance-for-Hospitals–Nursing-Homes–and-Other-Health-Care-Facilities—FDA-Public-Health-Advisory.pdf. Accessed April 28, 2020.
35. Friesen RM. Oxygen concentrators and the practice of anaesthesia. Can J Anaesth 1992;39:R80–4.
36. Westwood MM, Tieley W. Medical gases, their storage and delivery. Anaesth Intensive Care 2012;13:533–8.
37. National Fire Protection Association. Compressed Gases and Cryogenic Fluids Code (NFPA 55). Quincy (MA): 2020.
38. Das S, Chattopadhyay S, Bose P. The anaesthesia gas supply system. Indian J Anaesth 2013;57:489–99.
39. Malayaman SN, Mychaskiw G, Ehrenworth J. Medical gases: storage and supply. In: Ehrenworth J, Eisenkraft JB, Berry JM, editors. Anesthesia equipment: principles and applications. 2nd edition. Philadelphia: Elsevier Saunders; 2013. p. 3–24.
40. Srivastava U. Anaesthesia gas supply: gas cylinders. Indian J Anaesth 2013;57: 500–6.
41. Hart JR, Rubadou CB, editors. Health care facilities code handbook. Quincy (MA): National Fire Protection Association; 2018.
42. Hart JR. Medical gas and vacuum systems handbook. Quincy (MA): National Fire Protection Association; 2018.
43. ASTM B819-19, standard specification for seamless copper tube for medical gas systems. West Conshohocken (PA): ASTM International; 2019.
44. Evans F, Winbourne P. The health of our piped medical gas distribution center. APSF Newsl 1993;8. Available at: https://www.apsf.org/article/danger-seen-possible-from-contaminated-medical-gases/. Accessed April 28, 2020.
45. Stoller JK, Stefanak M, Orens D, et al. The hospital oxygen problem: an "O2K" problem. Respir Care 2000;45:300–5.
46. ISO 80601-2-13:2011, Medical electrical equipment-part 2-13: particular requirements for basic safety and essential performance of an anaesthetic workstation. Geneva (Switzerland): International Organization for Standardization; 2011.
47. Goode RL, Breen PH. Anesthesia machine and circuit: portal to the respiratory system. Anest Clin North Am 1998;16:1–28.
48. Taenzer AH, Kovatsis PG, Raessler KL. E-cylinder-powered mechanical ventilation may adversely impact anesthetic management and efficiency. Anesth Analg 2002;95:148–50.
49. Klemenzson GK, Perouansky M. Contemporary anesthesia ventilators incur a significant "oxygen cost. Can J Anaesth 2004;51:616–20.
50. Ritchie JR. A simple and reliable warning device for falling oxygen pressure. Br J Anaesth 1974;46:323.

51. Standards for basic anesthetic monitoring. Schaumburg (IL): American Society of Anesthesiologists; 2015. Available at: https://www.asahq.org/standards-and-guidelines/standards-for-basic-anesthetic-monitoring. Accessed April 28, 2020.

52. 2016 Medical gas container-closure rule questions and answers: guidance for industry. Silver Springs (MD): Food and Drug Administration; 2017. Available at: https://www.fda.gov/media/102638/download. Accessed April 28, 2020.

53. CGA P-15. Filling of industrial and medical non-flammable compressed gas cylinders. Arlington (VA): Compressed Gas Association, Inc; 2016.

54. Feeley TW, McClelland KJ, Malhotra IV. The hazards of bulk oxygen delivery systems. Lancet 1975;7922:1416–8.

55. Botney R, Gaba DM. Human factors issues in monitoring. In: Blitt CD, Hines RL, editors. Monitoring in anesthesia and critical care medicine. 3rd edition. New York: Churchill Livingstone; 1995. p. 23–54.

56. Botney R, Gaba DM, Howard SK. Anesthesiologist performance during a simulated loss of pipeline oxygen. Anest 1993;79:A1118.

57. Lorraway PG, Savoldelli GL, Joo HS, et al. Management of simulated oxygen supply failure: is there a gap in the curriculum? Anesth Analg 2006;102:865–7.

58. Berkenstadt H, Ezri T, Sidi A, et al. Management of simulated oxygen supply failure and expiratory valve malfunction: is there a curriculum gap? Simulation in Healthcare: The Journal of the Society for Simulation in Healthcare 2007;2:56.

59. Merry AF, Weller JM, Robinson BJ, et al. A simulation design for research evaluating safety innovations in anaesthesia. Anaesthesia 2008;63:1349–57.

60. Waldrop WB, Murray DJ, Boulet JR, et al. Management of anesthesia equipment failure: a simulation-based resident skill assessment. Anesth Analg 2009;109:426–33.

61. Mudumbai SC, Fanning R, Howard SK, et al. Use of medical simulation to explore equipment failures and human-machine interactions in anesthesia machine pipeline supply crossover. Anesth Analg 2010;110:1292–6.

62. Botney R, Berenholtz SM, Seagull FJ. Introduction to patient safety. In: Young VL, Botney R, editors. Patient safety in plastic surgery. St Louis (MO): Quality Medical Publishing; 2009. p. 3–42.

63. Kacmarek RM. Central oxygen delivery systems: a disaster waiting to happen? Respir Care 2000;45:299.

UNITED STATES POSTAL SERVICE ® — Statement of Ownership, Management, and Circulation (All Periodicals Publications Except Requester Publications)

1. Publication Title	2. Publication Number	3. Filing Date
ANESTHESIOLOGY CLINICS	000 - 275	9/18/2020

4. Issue Frequency	5. Number of Issues Published Annually	6. Annual Subscription Price
MAR, JUN, SEP, DEC	4	$364.00

7. Complete Mailing Address of Known Office of Publication (Not printer) (Street, city, county, state, and ZIP+4®)

ELSEVIER INC.
230 Park Avenue, Suite 800
New York, NY 10169

Contact Person
Malathi Samayan

Telephone (Include area code)
91-44-4299-4507

8. Complete Mailing Address of Headquarters or General Business Office of Publisher (Not printer)

ELSEVIER INC.
230 Park Avenue, Suite 800
New York, NY 10169

9. Full Names and Complete Mailing Addresses of Publisher, Editor, and Managing Editor (Do not leave blank)

Publisher (Name and complete mailing address)

DOLORES MELONI, ELSEVIER INC.
1600 JOHN F KENNEDY BLVD. SUITE 1800
PHILADELPHIA, PA 19103-2899

Editor (Name and complete mailing address)

JOANNA COLLETT, ELSEVIER INC.
1600 JOHN F KENNEDY BLVD. SUITE 1800
PHILADELPHIA, PA 19103-2899

Managing Editor (Name and complete mailing address)

PATRICK MANLEY, ELSEVIER INC.
1600 JOHN F KENNEDY BLVD. SUITE 1800
PHILADELPHIA, PA 19103-2899

10. Owner (Do not leave blank. If the publication is owned by a corporation, give the name and address of the corporation immediately followed by the names and addresses of all stockholders owning or holding 1 percent or more of the total amount of stock. If not owned by a corporation, give the names and addresses of the individual owners. If owned by a partnership or other unincorporated firm, give its name and address as well as those of each individual owner. If the publication is published by a nonprofit organization, give its name and address.)

Full Name	Complete Mailing Address
WHOLLY OWNED SUBSIDIARY OF REED/ELSEVIER, US HOLDINGS	1600 JOHN F KENNEDY BLVD. SUITE 1800 PHILADELPHIA, PA 19103-2899

11. Known Bondholders, Mortgagees, and Other Security Holders Owning or Holding 1 Percent or More of Total Amount of Bonds, Mortgages, or Other Securities. If none, check box ☑ None

Full Name	Complete Mailing Address
N/A	

12. Tax Status (For completion by nonprofit organizations authorized to mail at nonprofit rates) (Check one)
The purpose, function, and nonprofit status of this organization and the exempt status for federal income tax purposes:
☒ Has Not Changed During Preceding 12 Months
☐ Has Changed During Preceding 12 Months (Publisher must submit explanation of change with this statement)

PS Form **3526**, July 2014 (Page 1 of 4 (see instructions page 4)) PSN 7530-01-000-9931 PRIVACY NOTICE: See our privacy policy on www.usps.com.

---

13. Publication Title		14. Issue Date for Circulation Data Below	
Anesthesiology Clinics		JUNE 2020	

15. Extent and Nature of Circulation			Average No. Copies Each Issue During Preceding 12 Months	No. Copies of Single Issue Published Nearest to Filing Date
a. Total Number of Copies (Net press run)			220	176
b. Paid Circulation (By Mail and Outside the Mail)	(1)	Mailed Outside-County Paid Subscriptions Stated on PS Form 3541 (Include paid distribution above nominal rate, advertiser's proof copies, and exchange copies)	79	68
	(2)	Mailed In-County Paid Subscriptions Stated on PS Form 3541 (Include paid distribution above nominal rate, advertiser's proof copies, and exchange copies)	0	0
	(3)	Paid Distribution Outside the Mails Including Sales Through Dealers and Carriers, Street Vendors, Counter Sales, and Other Paid Distribution Outside USPS®	94	73
	(4)	Paid Distribution by Other Classes of Mail Through the USPS (e.g. First-Class Mail®)	0	0
c. Total Paid Distribution (Sum of 15b (1), (2), (3), and (4))		►	173	141
d. Free or Nominal Rate Distribution (By Mail and Outside the Mail)	(1)	Free or Nominal Rate Outside-County Copies included on PS Form 3541	29	18
	(2)	Free or Nominal Rate In-County Copies Included on PS Form 3541	0	0
	(3)	Free or Nominal Rate Copies Mailed at Other Classes Through the USPS (e.g. First-Class Mail)	0	0
	(4)	Free or Nominal Rate Distribution Outside the Mail (Carriers or other means)	0	0
e. Total Free or Nominal Rate Distribution (Sum of 15d (1), (2), (3) and (4))		►	29	18
f. Total Distribution (Sum of 15c and 15e)		►	202	159
g. Copies not Distributed (See Instructions to Publishers #4 (page 83))		►	18	17
h. Total (Sum of 15f and g)		►	220	176
i. Percent Paid (15c divided by 15f times 100)			85.64%	88.67%

* If you are claiming electronic copies, go to line 16 on page 3. If you are not claiming electronic copies, skip to line 17 on page 3.

16. Electronic Copy Circulation		Average No. Copies Each Issue During Preceding 12 Months	No. Copies of Single Issue Published Nearest to Filing Date
a. Paid Electronic Copies	►		
b. Total Paid Print Copies (Line 15c) + Paid Electronic Copies (Line 16a)	►		
c. Total Print Distribution (Line 15f) + Paid Electronic Copies (Line 16a)	►		
d. Percent Paid (Both Print & Electronic Copies) (16b divided by 16c × 100)	►		

☒ I certify that 50% of all my distributed copies (electronic and print) are paid above a nominal price.

17. Publication of Statement of Ownership

☒ If the publication is a general publication, publication of this statement is required. Will be printed in the DECEMBER 2020 issue of this publication. ☐ Publication not required.

18. Signature and Title of Editor, Publisher, Business Manager, or Owner		Date
Malathi Samayan - Distribution Controller	*Malathi Samayan*	9/18/2020

I certify that all information furnished on this form is true and complete. I understand that anyone who furnishes false or misleading information on this form or who omits material or information requested on the form may be subject to criminal sanctions (including fines and imprisonment) and/or civil sanctions (including civil penalties).

PS Form **3526**, July 2014 (Page 3 of 4) PRIVACY NOTICE: See our privacy policy on www.usps.com.

Moving?

Make sure your subscription moves with you!

To notify us of your new address, find your **Clinics Account Number** (located on your mailing label above your name), and contact customer service at:

Email: journalscustomerservice-usa@elsevier.com

800-654-2452 (subscribers in the U.S. & Canada)
314-447-8871 (subscribers outside of the U.S. & Canada)

Fax number: 314-447-8029

Elsevier Health Sciences Division
Subscription Customer Service
3251 Riverport Lane
Maryland Heights, MO 63043

*To ensure uninterrupted delivery of your subscription, please notify us at least 4 weeks in advance of move.